WHAT I CAN SEE FOR YOU!

What I Can See For You!

When Ruth Barrett seeks treatment for a minor eye infection, she has no conception of the rapid decline in health that her prescribed treatment will promote or the desperate struggle that must follow before she can regain her health.

This book is written as a warning to all those who value their health; of the side effects of modern medicine that can be worse than the treatment and the inherent dangers of combining New Age and alternative medicine without a full and knowledgeable understanding of their devastating potential.

What I Can See For You!

Ruth Barrett

Writers Club Press

San Jose New York Lincoln Shanghai

Published by Writers Club Press
an imprint of iUniverse.com, Inc.

For information address:
iUniverse.com, Inc.
620 North 48th Street
Suite 201
Lincoln, NE 68504-3467
www.iuniverse.com

ISBN: 0-595-13123-9

Printed in the United States of America

Dedication

Dedicated to the memory of David, my beloved husband.

Introduction

Good health and a long life are the hopes of nearly everyone. A vast amount of effort is spent by all civilised societies to help people achieve this. Great advances have taken place over the last few hundred years, but there is still a very long way to go....

This book is written as a witness as to what can go wrong with "medicine" in the last decade of the 20th century as it is currently practised and made available to the population.

There are many "alternative" treatments available which have in some instances outstanding success. The temptation to seek these cures increases dramatically when the level of distress due to an illness becomes acute.

When conventional medicine doesn't seem to help then other alternatives become attractive, but what happens when they are mixed? Because so little is generally understood about this, the answer is perhaps nobody knows. The dangers can be immense but there is no mechanism to find out at the moment.

Ruth Barrett felt that as she only had one body for this life, it was a good idea to look after it. If an ailment inflicted itself on her then a cure should be found and taken until all was well....

Unfortunately the side effects of modem medicine can be worse than the affliction. In Ruth's case curing a simple eye infection gave rise to becoming vulnerable to additional afflictions which were not immediately understood and the wrong cures were offered leading to a rapidly worsening situation. What happened next describes a long battle to overcome all these difficulties plus the effect of mixing various cures

Everyone has a right to the best health care they can get, but how can one be guided through all the conventional and unconventional treatments possible. This guidance is vital but just not available. Many more will find out the hard way, like Ruth, until this dilemma is solved (if it ever is!).

This book is written in the hope that others will read it and learn that common sense and caution are needed when seeking an urgently needed cure. The mentors are few and far between so good luck is perhaps needed more than good judgement (because that is incredibly hard to achieve with confidence).

Tim Moore
July, 1996.

CHAPTER I

In the autumn of 1968 1 consulted a lady clairvoyant. She was in fact a psychometrist, i.e. a person who holds an article belonging to you and then after picking up your vibrations is able to see your past, present and future.

Circumstances at the time had led me to contact her, although I had never consulted any psychic or medium before, even though I am a little psychic myself, having had precognitive dreams and glimpses of precognition in the form of pictures flashing before my eyes and other experiences. Ironically, I had always been apprehensive of the fact that they might tell me something it was better I didn't hear.

I had picked her name at random out of the adverts I saw in the magazine 'Prediction' and made an appointment to see her. She lived in a flat in the West End of London and the door was opened by a rather plump middle-aged lady with auburn hair. She led me into the sitting room where we both sat down, "Give me an article to hold," she said.

I gave her my wrist watch and sat patiently while she closed her eyes and concentrated for a short time. She then said enthusiastically, "I'm picking up your vibrations."

She began her reading, telling me many things, including the fact that I would have dealings with a publisher in the future.

Suddenly, however, in the midst of the reading, a man's disembodied voice bellowed into my right ear, "What I can see for you!" I had never heard a spirit voice before and I was totally stunned.

The psychometrist went on with her reading completely unaware of what I had just experienced and I left without telling her. However, I regarded it as an ominous warning at the time, and after the terrible ordeal I was to go through years later it proved, indeed, to be so. I was to remember what that wretched and, in my opinion, mischievous spirit bellowed in my right ear over and over again.

Because of that experience, however, instead of being completely put off by psychics, I went on to consult a few more, but I was more discerning in my choice. I only consulted clairvoyants who I knew had good reputations, and among them was a very genteel, silver-haired lady in her sixties. She lived near Marble Arch in London and she called herself a natural clairvoyant. "I can see spirits and they tell me things," she said.

I mentioned that I had recently consulted the psychometrist, giving her name and telling her what had happened during the reading. She shook her head sadly, saying, "You know I have people coming here who have been frightened out of their wits by what she's told them."

I could believe it. Mediums keep telling us that there are many souls trapped in a kind of limbo, unaware that they are dead and capable of exercising negative influences. And a year or two later I was to read in an article about the psychometrist in question that she regularly used a ouija board to contact spirits, and, because of that very dangerous practice I am convinced that she had surrounded herself with spirits who were indeed malevolent.

The same clairvoyant, went on to predict happenings which would later come to pass. She also surprised me at the time by saying, "Writing is for you," which again I dismissed as something that couldn't possibly be correct.

Soon afterwards, I consulted the famous medium and clairvoyant Douglas Johnson and he predicted the same thing. As soon as I entered his Chelsea house and walked into his sitting room he said, "I must tell you before we start that I saw writing big, the moment you came in through the door. I saw success."

"But I can't make up anything," I replied in amazement.

"Then something will happen that you will write about," he replied. "It's your own story."

His prediction came to pass, for, many years later, something did happen which prompted me to write this book—a chain of events that tested me to my physical and mental limits which I felt lucky to survive. But I did survive and this is my story.

It all began innocently enough on one cold, wintry day in March 1982. I went to the casualty department of a famous eye hospital—to the branch in Holborn which is now closed. I had noticed a tiny lump on the inside of my lower right eyelid. It didn't affect me in the least, but being somewhat over-anxious I wanted to know what it was. A friend who had lost an eye in childhood had recommended me to the hospital and they had been 'looking after' him for years.

On that fateful day I walked up to the nurse in reception and told her about the lump. She felt my lower lid and then said, "Take a seat in the waiting room and we will call you when we are ready for you."

I went into the tiny, very crowded, waiting room and sat there for what seemed like hours until a nurse called out my name.

I followed her into a large room where the doctors were treating their patients. She pulled down my lower lid and said, "The doctor will do it for you now."

"Will he?" I asked in surprise, after all I had only gone there to ease my mind and find out the nature of the lump.

She tested my eyesight which was a routine measure, and then told me to go back into the waiting room and wait until I was called again.

It wasn't long before I heard my name being called and once again I went back into the room.

A rather sullen nurse led me to what looked like a dentist's chair and told me to sit down. "The doctor will be with you shortly," she said.

I sat there wondering what to expect when, suddenly, from behind a panel I heard a doctor say to a patient, "You've got no retina." He sounded shocked by the discovery.

Soon afterwards, however, the same doctor breezed into the room from behind the panel. He was dark haired and very young looking and he babbled on excitedly to the nurse, saying, "I've never seen anyone without a retina before."

He went over to the basin to wash his hands and then came over to me. He stood behind my chair while the unsmiling, seemingly unfeeling nurse held my hand. It was just my luck to have her I mused, all the other nurses were friendly and helpful.

The doctor then began doing something with my right eye and I blinked.

"Don't blink!" the young doctor bellowed. "You've got a needle in your eye. I'm freezing it."

"How irresponsible," I muttered to myself, thinking that he should have warned me what he was about to do.

A minute or two later he began probing in my eyelid and the pain was so excruciating that I moaned and groaned and gripped the nurse's hand tightly.

"So much for him freezing it," I said to myself.

Throughout my ordeal, however, the young doctor kept babbling on about his last patient. He couldn't seem to get over the fact that he had seen a person without a retina and I felt like telling him to "Shut up" and just concentrate on what he was doing to me, while the nurse just glared at me the whole time. She showed no sympathy whatsoever.

After he had finished the 'operation', the doctor said jauntily, "It might bleed a little," and off he went to wash his hands in the basin. The nurse put a cotton wool pad over my eye, securing it with sticky tape.

"Come back if you have any problems," said the young doctor as he walked out of the room.

Problems! My God! That tiny so-called operation was to lead to my going through years of suffering. One problem led to another, and the combination of horrors that occurred I may not have been able to survive.

As soon as the nurse had secured my cotton wool eye pad, I got up from my seat and promptly stumbled and fell. I had lost my sense of balance. One of the nurses came to my aid and said, "It's only to be expected."

I was then handed a card and led to the reception desk. I showed the card to the lady at the desk and she said, "Go to the pharmacy. They will give you some ointment and tell you what you have to do."

I groped my way to the pharmacy and handed the card to the lady behind the counter. She gave me some ointment called chioramphenicol which, I found out later, was a very powerful germ killer.

"Take the covering off after six hours," she said. "Don't leave it on any longer, and squeeze the ointment into the eye three times a day for three days and then leave it off."

I walked rather unsteadily back to where I had promised to meet my husband, across some very busy roads. A colleague of his saw me and exclaimed, "What have they done to you!"

"Oh it's nothing serious," I replied confidently.

Fortunately, I was driven the rest of the way home, and after six hours, following their instructions implicitly, I took off the cotton wool pad. My eye was badly bruised and swollen, but I knew it would soon heal. I could detect, however, a tiny slit on the inside of my lower lid where the doctor had probed, but thankfully it wasn't very noticeable. I continued to do as I was told and I squeezed the ointment into my eye every day for three days. Not for one moment did I think that anything could possibly go wrong.

A few weeks passed without my noticing anything untoward happening, but I became a little frightened when I thought I saw flashes before my eyes as I lay awake in the dark, so back I went to the casualty department of the eye hospital.

I told the receptionist what was troubling me and was once again told to wait in the waiting room. Soon, a nurse came and took me into the treatment room. She put drops into my eyes to widen the pupils so that the doctor could see behind them. I was then required to wait half an hour while the drops took effect. "Your vision will be blurred," she warned.

On that occasion I saw another young doctor. He was tall and fair and very charming. He looked carefully into both of my eyes with a bright light and then said, "I can't see anything wrong, but you've recently had an operation on your eye and things take a long time to settle down." I left feeling much happier.

However, as the weeks passed my eye became more and more irritated. I used Optrex in an effort to soothe it, but it was becoming evident that things were not going to settle down.

That summer, I travelled abroad visiting, among other places, Hungary, Czechoslovakia and Austria. And, apart from the irritation in my eye, I felt very well and extremely happy.

For the past year I had suffered from inflammation of the stomach and had been obliged to take libraxin tablets before each meal. But it had all cleared up by then. My GP had referred me to St Thomas' Hospital after she had failed to help me. She had given me the wonder drug 'Targamet' which cures ulcers. But, after an endoscopy and a barium meal test at the hospital, the lady specialist said, "You haven't got an ulcer but there is inflammation. I'm going to prescribe for you a harmless drug called libraxin. It relaxes the gut. Take one before each meal and leave it off when you think you can. It may take a year." It had taken a year.

She was indeed a very thorough specialist. I liked her very much and I saw her once or twice after that, but she was pregnant at the time and was obliged to take time off to have her baby. Alas, in her place I had seen a young male specialist and all he had to say to me, with considerable irritation, was, "Go home and alter your ways. There's nothing we can do for you here!"

"When I did see the lady specialist again I told her what he had said to me, and she wasn't very pleased.

The week after I returned from abroad, a very red, nasty looking lump appeared on my lower eyelid. I kept bathing it with Optrex but the lump would not go away. So once again I was obliged to return to the eye hospital.

I was given the routine eye test and again told to wait in the waiting room until called to see the doctor. I didn't have to wait long before being called and I went into the treatment area where two doctors were sitting alongside one another, both treating patients. The first doctor to be free was a heavily built man in his thirties. He had a trainee doctor sitting behind him.

He sat for a moment or two looking at my notes and then he asked me to put my chin on the apparatus called a slit lamp which was in front of me. He looked into both eyes with a light and then exclaimed, "My God! He's made a mess of it!"

He turned to the trainee doctor and gave a deep sigh, then, turning to me he said, "You've got an infection in the eye which is very difficult to get rid of."

I was momentarily too shocked to speak and I just stared at him. I then quickly glanced at the doctor and his patient sitting alongside us. They had obviously heard what the doctor had said to me and they were both looking at me with concern on their faces.

The bearded doctor then turned to the trainee doctor and asked, "Do you remember the other patient we had?"

He nodded sympathetically.

I just couldn't believe it. I had carried out all their instructions to the letter after the wretched operation. So what had gone wrong?

The doctor then stared into my eyes and said, "It's up to you. Do you want to leave it or do you want to go through it all?"

"Of course I want it healed. You can't leave an infection in my eye. I have trouble with it every day," I replied immediately, thinking it was a stupid question to ask.

"Very well," he said, "I will give you some antibiotics. You are to take them for three months. You won't notice any improvement until after the first month because the infection is so deep-seated. After that it should improve. But you must take the full course."

I nodded; I was prepared to do anything. "Will it cure it?" I asked anxiously.

"If that doesn't, nothing will," he promptly replied.

I thanked the doctor and went to the pharmacy with my prescription. The antibiotic they gave me was a tetracycline. At that time I was totally unaware of the dangers of taking too many antibiotics, especially the tetracyclines which destroy the natural bowel flora. The doctor who prescribed the massive dosage of antibiotics should have warned me, but he didn't and the consequences proved disastrous.

However, after I had taken the antibiotics for a month I saw no improvement whatsoever. In fact, things seemed to be getting worse. Both eyes were now affected. They felt irritated all the time with big red bubbles on both my swollen lower lids. The upper lids were also inflamed and swollen. They wept continually and the inflammation of my right eye had penetrated as far down as my lower cheek.

So, after six weeks I went back to the eye hospital, deliberately picking the same day so as to see the same specialist. He was alone when I entered the clinic, the other doctor had gone to the canteen.

I sat opposite him and naturally expected him to behave as he had done before. But his whole attitude towards me had changed. He had recognised me and clearly didn't want to see me again.

"My eyes are in an awful state," I told him. "Both eyes are affected. They are red, swollen and irritated and they continually weep."

He looked into both eyes. "Well done," he snapped coldly. "You've got rid of the infection." He had completely ignored what I had told him and I couldn't believe it.

He was, it seemed, just about to dismiss me when I pleaded, "But I've just told you what trouble I am having with them." I felt in desperate need of help.

"Don't tell me my job, "he said angrily. "I'm telling you I can find nothing wrong with them." He sat glaring at me. And because he had turned out to be such a monster I didn't know what to do, so I just asked, "Well, shall I stop taking the antibiotics?"

"No, you'd better finish the course to make sure the infection doesn't come back," he replied.

"But I'm still having so much trouble with them," I continued to plead.

"Well, if they continually run, then perhaps the tear ducts are blocked," he snapped, his eyes blazing. "The nurse will see to that." He hastily wrote on a piece of paper and thrusting his hand out he said impatiently, "Give this to the nurse in the next room."

I took the piece of paper and went into the adjoining room. I gave it to the nurse and she asked me to sit on the chair. She then inserted water into the tiny holes on the insides of both eyes to test if my tear ducts were blocked. Clearly they weren't.

She wrote on the piece of paper and gave it to me, sending me back to see the doctor who was by that time treating another patient. I waited until he had finished and when he was ready to see me again I handed him the piece of paper and he said impatiently, "Well there's nothing wrong with your tear ducts."

But when I once again protested that I was in need of help he stood up and shouted, "Get out. Go on get out!"

I just looked at him in horror. He had no cause for such behaviour but I didn't argue further. Tears welled up in my eyes and I got up and walked slowly to the door, passing a lady patient who had overheard everything. "What a way to be treated," she whispered.

When I reached the door, I turned and I took a last look at the doctor who had treated me so badly. Our eyes met and I heard him whisper, "Perhaps she'll report me."

The wretched man deserved it, but I didn't want to waste my time.

A week later I went again to the eye hospital. It happened to be on the same day of the week, but I was determined not to see the same doctor. Fortunately, when it was my turn the doctor had left the clinic so there was no problem. I saw his colleague.

"What can I do for you?" he asked, politely but rather coldly. He had read my notes, so I simply told him everything I was experiencing and he looked carefully into both eyes.

"You've got blebepharious in both eyes," he said matter of factly and he began writing out a prescription.

"Has the infection gone into my right eye?" I asked.

"I don't know anything about an infection," he said, although it must have been written in my notes. Nevertheless, I could see from his attitude that he didn't intend to be drawn any further on the subject, so I left it at that.

As he was handing me the prescription the bearded doctor walked into the room. He just stood and stared at us. The fact that I was being given a prescription had dumbfounded him. I got up from my seat and glared at him. "She won't come to see me again," he mouthed to himself.

He was right. If he couldn't see anything wrong with my eyes when they were in such an appalling state, then he wasn't only unbelievably rude he was totally incompetent.

The prescription was for chloramphenicol, which I was told to rub in each night. The ointment was very harsh and it made my lids swell up. I looked an awful sight and I was too embarrassed to go out.

For weeks I rubbed in the ointment, but things didn't appear to be getting any better. I was beginning to despair that they would ever heal and look normal again. Apart from their appearance, I would wake up in the night with burning pain in my right eye and I would bathe it with Optrex to try and sootht it.

After my experiences at the hospital I felt it was time I consulted a specialist privately, so I telephoned one I had seen advertised in the Yellow Pages. A lady answered.

"Is it possible to see the specialist privately?" I asked.

"I'm afraid my husband is away at the moment. What is the problem?" she replied.

I told her what had happened and where I had been treated.

"I can give you the name and telephone number of a consultant at the eye hospital you mentioned," she replied.

"Yes please," I said eagerly.

I took down the number and telephoned the consultant as soon as I could. His secretary answered. I told her my problems and asked if it was possible to make an appointment to see the consultant privately.

"I'll phone you back when I've arranged a time with him," she said.

She telephoned about an hour later. "The consultant will see you tomorrow if you could come to the clinic in the main building. Be there at 2.30 p.m. The notes from the casualty department of the other branch will be shunted over. It is called the Clinic of Tropical Diseases," she said.

"What!" I exclaimed.

"Yes I know, it's a terrible name," she laughed.

I expressed my gratitude to her and told her I would definitely be there.

I turned up early for my appointment and found the huge main building almost deserted.

I made my way to the Clinic of Tropical Diseases and reported to the receptionist. She was a middle-aged lady and she snapped, "You're early. There's no one here yet."

She began looking for my notes, but couldn't find any.

"I haven't got your notes," she said irritably. "Go to the reception office in the main hall and ask for them there, then bring them back to me."

I made my way to the main hall and asked the receptionist if she had my notes. She told me to sit on a bench while she searched for them.

I was alone on the bench until a woman came and sat down beside me. I glanced at her and the poor woman seemed terribly embarrassed, for she had a very unsightly growth at the top of her nose, close to her eye. Her eye was also bloodshot and swollen.

"What happened to you?" I asked.

"Oh, they gave me treatment that was too strong for me," she replied calmly. "I've come here for a second opinion. At the other hospital they said they couldn't cure it."

"Why not?" I asked, feeling very sorry for her.

"Yes, why not," she replied with a fighting spirit.

She was certainly coping better than I was. Because of my unsightly appearance I was becoming very emotional.

Eventually, I was given my notes which I took back to the disagreeable receptionist. By then the rows of benches in the waiting area were filling up, and soon hundreds seemed to be milling around.

The afternoon session was about to begin. Each patient was called in turn and eventually I heard my name being called by the consultant himself.

He led me into a large room which was crowded with doctors and patients.

He sat himself down by his desk, which was near the entrance and indicated where I should sit. There was a gentleman observer sitting next to him.

I sat on the chair he had indicated, and no sooner had I done so the consultant's loud voice boomed out, "Don't sit there, it's next to a radiator." He turned to the gentleman sitting beside him and roared with laughter while the whole room fell silent, probably wondering what had precipitated such an outburst from him. It was an ominous start and my heart started to thump. We hadn't started and I felt he was already making fun of me.

I moved my chair away from the radiator and nearer to his desk.

"I know what's wrong with you. You're emotionally disturbed," he said loudly. "That should be treated first." And he again turned to the gentleman sitting beside him and laughed, but the gentleman didn't turn his way. He kept his eyes fixed on mine as if to tell me that he too found the consultant's behaviour abhorrent.

The consultant then rapidly turned over the pages of my notes and exclaimed, "My God! I'll have to tighten things up there." I was of the same opinion but I kept quiet.

He got up from his seat and said curtly, "Come with me." I was taken into a small adjoining room where he did thoroughly examine my eyes. But when it was over and we were walking back to his desk he said sneeringly, "And she wanted to see me privately."

As soon as we were both seated again, he leaned over to me and whispered, "You haven't got any disease…nothing that will affect the eyesight anyway."

It was a relief to hear that.

"Have you had a swab taken?" he asked in a loud voice, quickly reverting to his former behaviour.

It seemed that the wretched man actually thought that he was impressing those around him by adopting that manner, but of course he was doing the exact opposite, judging by the look on their faces.

"No, I haven't had a swab taken," I answered.

He gave a sigh of exasperation and quickly wrote on a card. Handing it to me, he said, "Go over there, they'll do it for you." He pointed out the direction.

Before leaving, I asked rather boldly, "Aren't you going to give me any treatment?"

"No, I'm not going to give you any treatment," he said, and then he added, "your own doctor can. ..if he wants to."

"It's a she," I retorted as I walked out of the room, thankful that my ordeal was finally over.

I made my way to the room across the hall where they took the swab. They told me the results would be sent to my GP and I despaired, knowing very well that it would prove a waste of everyone's time.

I walked out of the hospital in a complete daze, eventually finding my way home. To behave the way that consultant did to a person who was clearly emotionally distraught was totally irresponsible. The consequences could have been fatal. I could easily have jumped in front of the first train—the thought did fleetingly pass through my mind. But believe it or not he wasn't the only consultant I was to encounter whose behaviour was beyond belief.

The following week I went again to the casualty department of the eye hospital in Holborn, but I went on a different day so as not to encounter either of the other two doctors. To my relief there was a lady specialist on that day and I desperately wanted to see her, but when my turn came she was, to my disappointment, attending to another patient in the adjoining room. The other doctor present was an extremely young-looking man but so languid. He appeared bored with everything.

I sat down opposite him. He had my notes in front of him and after glancing through them he looked into both my eyes with a bright light. Afterwards he shrugged his shoulders and said, "I can't see anything wrong with them."

Immediately I protested. I wasn't going to be dismissed that easily.

"I'll go and see if my colleague will see you," he said, and he went into the next room, returning immediately. "My colleague says she will see you as soon as she's finished with her patient," he said, again without showing any real interest.

The lady doctor came and sat down opposite me. She too was very young, pretty and extremely charming. She gave me a broad smile and I relaxed immediately. I wasn't used to that kind of treatment.

She read carefully through my notes and then said, "What did the consultant say? He teaches me."

Immediately I began telling her what had happened at the other clinic and how badly I felt the consultant had behaved towards me. She listened, with interest, to everything I said and didn't attempt to stop me. Her colleague, however, kept giving me threatening glances. But I couldn't stop, and at the end of the tirade she simply said, "It doesn't surprise me. Consultants think they are gods...but I want to be a consultant one day."

I hoped she would achieve her ambition.

I bent forward so that she could take a look at my eye and she said, glancing at her colleague, "You don't need a light to see what's wrong with the eye, you can tell by just looking at it." Turning to me, she said, "I'll give you some ointment that will soothe the eye. The ointment that you have been given is very harsh and I'll give you another fortnight of tetracycline. The doctor was right to give you tetracycline."

"But I've already taken months of it," I protested. I was already getting worried at the amount of antibiotics I had been obliged to take and at that time I wasn't even remotely aware of the dangers.

"Only a fortnight," she reassured me.

I reluctantly agreed to take them.

"Come and see me in a fortnight's time. I'm here every Wednesday," she said, showing her concern. It was the first time I had been asked to return to the hospital.

The ointment that she had given me quickly reduced the swelling, but they were nowhere near to being healed. The outer corner of the lower lid of my right eye was like a piece of dough, completely misshapen and I had lost my eyelashes. The lids of both my eyes were still badly inflamed and irritated and they wept profusely. I took to wearing dark glasses every time I went out.

In the end I saw my GP about the problem and asked for a referral letter to see a specialist at St Thomas' Hospital.

She pulled down the lower lid of my right eye and said, "Yes, it is still very red."

She asked me what ointments I had used and I told her. "I'll give you some drops," she said. "They burn for a short time. I use them for mine. My eyes feel very gritty in the night. They help a lot. They are called Opticrom."

But when I told her the length of time I had taken antibiotics she looked somewhat alarmed. "They take all the vitamins out of the system," she said with concern. "I'll give you a prescription for multivitamin tablets and I'll write a referral letter to St Thomas' Hospital."

I bitterly regretted not having gone there in the first place when I had discovered the lump. But now it was too late, the damage had been done. And I can see now that what was to follow would never have happened if it hadn't been for that disastrous so-called operation on my eye.

CHAPTER 2

On a few occasions I had visited the Spiritualist Church not far from home. I am a Christian and not a true Spiritualist, but I do believe that death is merely a transition into the spiritual world where we carry on where we leave off in progression. That we are all part of the Godhead and that love is the unifying force of the whole universe. And believing that all inspiration comes from the spiritual world I certainly believe in spiritual healing.

Spiritual healers were in attendance at the church on certain evenings each week and I had received healing from them. But one evening I decided to stay for the Evening of Clairvoyance. The medium was a silver-haired lady in her sixties. She had piercing eyes and a forthright manner.

There were only twenty people seated there and she went around every one in turn giving them clairvoyance. Somehow I felt she was avoiding me but, towards the end of the meeting, when she had spoken to almost everyone else she looked at me.

"And now for you," she said with a grimace. "I can see nothing but dark depression around you." She quickly turned away from me and then added, "We all have to go through it. I've gone through it myself. You are just paying back Karma."

I knew that Karma was the natural law of punishment for misdeeds in a past life—the law of cause and effect—if, of course, you believed in reincarnation, and she went on, "And when it's over, and it will be over, you will have more sympathy for other people's suffering."

I felt that I already had enough sympathy for other people's suffering, but perhaps I still had a lot to learn.

However, before moving on to another person she said quickly, "But underneath the dark depression it's golden."

At the end of the meeting I couldn't get away from the Spiritualist Church quick enough. Being already in a highly emotional state because of the condition of my eyes it was the last thing I wanted to hear. But she had said that it was golden underneath the dark depression and that was some consolation.

Not long after that experience I happened to be in Manchester for a few days with David, my husband, and walking through John Lewis, the big department store, I saw a man who was giving clairvoyance. He only charged £5 so I couldn't resist it. I asked for a consultation.

"I've been giving clairvoyance for thirty years," he told me.

I'm sure that was correct, but he only looked in his early forties. I found him to be an extremely personable man, very friendly and he turned out to be one of the best clairvoyants I have ever consulted. He used cards and I had to shuffle them again and again and he would lay them out on the table and tell me many things but, in the midst of the reading, he suddenly stopped, his face flushed and a look of horror came over it. He then said very slowly, "For several years life for you will be very difficult. If you had come to me years ago I still would have seen it." He paused, and then looking upwards he closed his eyes and prayed, "Please God may it be over," he said quietly.

It was yet another ominous warning of things to come, and I was again to remember what the wretched spirit voice had bellowed in my ear.

After a few weeks, however, the appointment came for me to attend St Thomas' Hospital. It had been a year since I had had the operation on my eye and I was no nearer getting them healed.

The specialist I saw was a Swedish lady in her forties. She was very charming and I liked her immediately. She asked me what had happened and I told her of my experiences at the other hospital. She was appalled.

"Who did the operation?" she demanded. "What's his name?"

"I don't know," I replied. I had never bothered to find out.

She took me into a cubicle and thoroughly examined my eyes. Afterwards she said angrily, "None of this should have happened." She was still furious.

We went back into the room and when we were both seated at her desk she asked, "What have you been using?"

I had brought the whole array of ointments with me and I laid them on the table.

"You've had some good stuff," she said as she picked up the chioraphemenicol. "I use this regularly on my eyes." Then, picking up the ointment that I had been given at the eye hospital to reduce the swelling, she said with disgust, "I wouldn't put that on my eye."

"Why not?" I asked somewhat surprised.

"They contain steroids," she replied. "They are very dangerous in prolonged use but I'm going to give you steroid drops. You are only to use them for a fortnight. That won't hurt you."

She wrote out a prescription for the drops and handing it to me said, "Come and see me in a fortnight's time."

I used the drops as I had been told to do and after a fortnight I went back to see the lady specialist.

She pulled down the lower lid of my right eye and said, "That's no good."

It was still badly inflamed. She then leaned over to me and whispered, "I shouldn't be telling you this but a friend of mine had inflammation in both eyes, just like you, but she lost all her eyelashes. She used chamomile teabags on her eyes and the inflammation cleared up and all her eyelashes came back. Just soak the bags in water for a short while, lie down and place the bags over the eyes for about a quarter of an hour a day. Try them."

"Yes, I will try them," I promised.

"But keep using the chioraphemenicol," she urged.

I couldn't wait to buy the chamomile teabags at the health shop and I used them straight away. They were fantastic. They brought out the inflammation, reduced the swelling and generally soothed the eyes. At last there were signs of improvement.

When next I saw the lady specialist she was pleased with my progress. "Have you had massage?" she enquired.

I shook my head.

"Come with me," she said.

I followed her into the small cubicle where, sitting opposite me, she began to press hard against my right eye with a tiny stick.

"Nothing's happening," she said, sounding somewhat disappointed.

She repeated the procedure and after waiting a few seconds she exclaimed, "Here it comes!"

She then began to probe the eyelid with a needle and when she had finished she urged, "Use the ointment for a few days after what I've done."

She had taken a tiny piece out of my lower right eyelid, but thankfully you'd have to look very close to see it.

By this time it was Christmas 1983 and the lady specialist went to Sweden for a holiday. In her place I saw the registrar, who was a tall, fair-haired, handsome young man. But he was extremely angry when he read my notes to find that I had been given steroid drops.

"It was only for a fortnight," I said, but he still wasn't very pleased.

However, after he had examined my eyes he conceded, "She did a very good job."

He went on to tell me to make a solution of bicarbonate of soda in hot water and after dipping cotton wool buds in the solution to run them across my lids.

"It's a very old and effective remedy for blebepharious, inflammation of the eyelids," he said. And he was shocked that I hadn't been given that simple piece of information before.

It turned out to be indeed a very effective remedy, and even to this day I regularly clean my eyes with a solution of bicarbonate of soda.

Just before Christmas 1983 I had seen a Harley Street specialist who was also a consultant at St Thomas' Hospital.

"I can still see the inflammation, but keep using the solution of bicarbonate of soda and it will go. If it doesn't go by March come and see me," he said.

I couldn't help telling him about the disgraceful way I had been treated by the young specialist and also the consultant at the eye hospital.

"They know what they have done," he replied simply. During the time I was having treatment at St Thomas' Hospital I saw the famous healer Ted Fricker.

There was an article in a newspaper about him and I wondered if it was possible to see him. I was thrilled to learn that he had a clinic in the West End of London which was listed in the directory. I rang the clinic and asked for an appointment. His wife answered and I was given an appointment for the following Wednesday at 2 p.m. There was a small fee of £10.

I found his waiting room packed with patients. I didn't know of course what they were suffering from but I knew he had a good reputation for curing cancer and I suspected that there were a lot of cancer patients waiting there.

However, the atmosphere in the waiting room was anything but gloomy. His wife acted as his receptionist and she was always chatty, very funny and she gave everyone a lift.

My problem I knew was trivial compared to some of the other patients but he had agreed to see me and I was emotionally very low, even more so after one unkind lady said to me, regarding my appearance, "You're ruined, I hope to God that it doesn't happen to me!"

It is incredible what lengths some people will go to just to be cruel.

However, when my turn came, I was ushered into Mr Fricker's room where I saw a genial, heavily built man sitting behind a large desk. He wore thick spectacles and he was much older than I had expected. He was in his seventies. He sat there looking well satisfied with life, which he had every right to be. He was indeed a very successful healer, which is a wonderful gift to have.

On his desk there was a lighted cigar and he picked it up and put it in his mouth, "What's the problem?" he asked.

Immediately I broke down and through my sobs I told him what had happened to my poor eyelids.

"I've had that before," he said nonchalantly. 'They'll heal. Take off your coat and sit on the stool."

As I began to take off my coat my wretched dark glasses fell out of the pocket.

"There you are," he said jovially, "that's God telling you that they will heal. Don't worry, they will heal."

I sat on a stool and he stood behind me. He put his massive hands over my eyes and pressed hard. My whole head seemed to vibrate. Apparently spirits spoke to him whilst he healed and he said, "The spirits are telling me that they will heal."

Eventually, of course, they did heal perfectly.

I went to him every few weeks for a couple of months. It was over Christmas time 1983 and his wife proudly showed me the Christmas card that Prince Charles had sent them. "He sends one every year," she said.

He regularly visited Chicago a few times a year and after one such visit he told me of the many cures he had had amongst the black population. "They expect to be cured and they are…but here," he said, shrugging his shoulders. I knew what he meant. We are such sceptics.

Alas, after Christmas and towards the end of my healing with him, I began having trouble with my stomach, but he once again assured me, "You are going to be fine."

CHAPTER 3

The trouble with my stomach and bowels began around the beginning of 1984. It started with a horrible feeling on the right side of my stomach and from then on I had sickness and diarrhoea practically every day.

One day I felt so ill with the sickness that I telephoned my GP.

"You don't need a visit," she said.

"But I feel so sick," I pleaded.

"Very well, I'll phone a chemist," she snapped, "and you can pick up a prescription from there. The drug will take away the sickness."

"Yes, that's fine," I replied gratefully.

She was already fed up with hearing from me. As far as she was concerned I had already become a nuisance with my continuing problem. But, after a few months with no sign of me getting better I went to see her again and she was forced to write another referral letter. I was referred to the gastro-intestinal clinic at St Thomas' Hospital. The one I had been referred to in 1981.

On my first visit I saw the consultant. He didn't have my notes, which displeased him, so I told him about the endoscopy and barium meal test I had in 1981 under the lady specialist.

"What did she diagnose?" he asked.

"She said that I had inflammation of the stomach," I replied.

"She was an excellent doctor and whatever she said the problem was then it was correct. Unfortunately she's not here any more, she's moved to another hospital," he said.

I was sorry to hear that.

"She gave me libraxin. They helped then but they don't seem to help any more," I told him. I had had some left over from the previous occasion and had tried taking them again, to no effect.

"The tablets I'm going to give you are much more powerful than libraxin," he said. "Come back in three weeks time and if it hasn't cleared up then you'll have to have tests."

The tablets were called stemetil and they did take away the nausea, but clearly all was not well with my stomach. I kept belching and it felt bloated and I still had the diarrhoea.

I didn't see the consultant on my next visit. Instead I saw the registrar, an oriental lady who was extremely rude. She didn't even bother to lift up her head to acknowledge me as I entered her consulting room, so I just sat down and waited while she hastily turned over the pages of my notes.

"You've had a lot of trouble with your stomach," she said impatiently and glared at me as if it was my fault. "You first came here in 1976."

(I had suffered from diarrhoea for six months, but after having an x-ray of my bowels it had just cleared up on its own. However, I had been told that I had a polyp.)

"The consultant gave you stemetil," she said. "Didn't that help?"

"Well it took away the nausea but my stomach is not right, it feels bloated and I keep belching and I still have the diarrhoea," I replied.

"Drink mint tea, that's good for wind," she said, obviously not taking me seriously.

"Can I have tests?" I asked. The consultant had said I could have tests if it hadn't cleared up.

"He says here that you don't need tests," she snapped.

I was getting so fed up with her rude behaviour that I began to show my Irritation with her. In the end I just got up from my seat and was about to walk out of the consulting room when she said hastily, 'Very well, you can have a urine and blood test."

My walking out on her had so shocked her that her attitude changed dramatically and she quickly signed the necessary forms and handed them to me.

"Send the results to me," I demanded angrily.

"We don't send the results to patients," she said apologetically.

"Send them to me," I repeated.

"Very well, I'll do that," she said meekly.

I then walked out of the door slamming it behind me. If I had been begging for charity I could not have been treated worse.

Two weeks later I had a letter from St Thomas' Hospital in which it stated that my blood and urine tests were normal.

However, my condition was getting steadily worse. My stomach didn't feel right, I had a vacuum feeling in it and it always felt bloated, plus the fact that I had nausea and sickness most days.

I had made another appointment to see a specialist at St Thomas' Hospital, but the night before my appointment I had the most terrible pain in the pit of my stomach and I was obliged to go to the toilet about fifteen times.

In the morning I managed to get some imodium tablets from the chemist and the diarrhoea stopped but I felt very weak. Fortunately, David was able to drive me to the hospital for my afternoon appointment. When I arrived I was told that I would again be seeing the registrar, but I adamantly refused to see the woman. Instead I saw a young, dark-haired gentleman who turned out to be friendly and helpful. He examined me thoroughly.

"I can't see any inflammation in your back passage," he said afterwards, "but there is a little mucous."

"I've taken imodium," I told him.

"Good. That's what I would have given you," he replied. "Take them for three days and then stop."

"Please can I have another endoscopy?" I pleaded.

"I don't see the point," he said, shaking his head. "You've already had one. I'll give you maxolon for your sickness."

The maxolon tablets helped, but they weren't getting to the root of the problem and when I saw the doctor a few weeks later and told him I was no better he relented and arranged for another endoscopy.

The endoscopy took place three weeks later, but unlike the previous occasion I wasn't given an injection to put me to sleep. They did give me an injection but it was just to relax me. I was fully conscious the whole time and I found it an ordeal. A tube with a light at the end called a gastro scope was put down my throat and the nurse held me down while I retched the whole time. "You're doing well," she kept repeating. The doctor was, of course, seated at the monitor observing everything throughout my ordeal, which probably only lasted about ten minutes, but it seemed an eternity to me and it was a tremendous relief when it was over.

I then sat in the waiting room, along with a few other patients, awaiting the results of the test.

About fifteen minutes later in walked the doctor who had taken the test. He came over to me and said quietly, "There's no disease—no cancers."

"Well that's good news," I replied. Thinking I might have the same trouble as before, I asked, "Is there any inflammation?"

"There's a little, but at the bottom of the gut, nothing much," he replied, and that was that.

I was given an appointment for a fortnight's time, so that the specialist could go over the results with me, and on that occasion I saw yet another doctor. I can't remember the reason why I wasn't able to see my usual one.

Whilst I was waiting to be seen by the doctor, a nurse desperately tried to get a rather quietly spoken woman to see the doctor in question. But she was adamant in refusing to see him. "He doesn't talk to you he shouts at you," she told the nurse. "I'm definitely not going to see him. I can well do without that." And she didn't see him.

I knew I was about to be seen by him and when my name was called I walked slowly into his consulting room expecting the worst.

"Sit down," he commanded in a loud, booming voice.

He was a young Australian doctor and it soon became evident that he couldn't behave in any other way.

"There's nothing wrong with your stomach," he bellowed. "The slight inflammation at the bottom of the gut is natural in everyone."

I didn't have the strength to argue with him and I just left the hospital, still nowhere nearer to finding the answer to my problems.

That summer, because my husband was in Los Angeles with the Royal Opera House for three weeks, I decided to travel to Los Angeles and join him. I had been to Los Angeles before in 1979 and enjoyed it immensely; I had also visited San Francisco and New York.

At the end of the tour we decided to travel by coach the whole width of the country from Los Angeles to New York. We travelled through Nevada, Colorado and Kentucky, ending up in Washington and then New York. It was another unforgettable journey and I kept going by taking maxolon tablets before each meal to stop me feeling sick. I love visiting America and I hope to go back there again in the not too distant future. Especially wonderful was flying over the Grand Canyon in a light aeroplane—the blend of colours and the immense size of it was breathtaking.

When I returned home my condition continued to deteriorate. I had frequent throat infections for which I was required to take even more antibiotics. On one occasion I went to see my GP because I had big red lumps inside my mouth and nasty sores on the corners of my mouth.

"You've got a fungus infection," she said. "That's why we don't give too many antibiotics."

She prescribed ten days' supply of nystatin, an effective drug which kills fungus infections. Later on, however, I was to become very familiar with that particular drug. She also prescribed oral nystatin to kill the thrush infection in my mouth.

After taking the course prescribed, the sores at the comers of my mouth cleared up and the lumps disappeared, but the other symptoms remained and because of my continuing downward spiral of ill-health I went again to see my GP and asked if I could have a second opinion at another hospital. She referred me to another hospital in South London.

On the day of my appointment my stomach felt horrible and I had the most severe diarrhoea. I had become a physical wreck, weak and exhausted.

The consultant questioned me thoroughly, but very matter of factly. He seemed very cold. I was then asked to go into the next room where a young doctor examined me. Meanwhile, the consultant spoke to my husband.

After the examination I went back into the consultant's room.

"The doctor can find nothing wrong with you and I am of the opinion that it's all emotional. I'm referring you to a psychiatrist," he told me.

He was hopelessly wrong. My illness was physical, but he was totally unaware of it. And because, at that time, I too was in the dark as to the true nature of my illness I could only comply.

"Which hospital would you like to attend?" he asked.

"St Thomas'," I answered, "because it's more convenient for me."

I was given another appointment.

Christmas came and passed and in January 1985 I was given an appointment to see a psychiatrist at St Thomas' Hospital.

The day I went to the hospital for my appointment I felt so ill and emotionally drained that I could barely lift my head to speak to anyone.

Firstly, I saw a junior doctor who took down all the essential details. I was then asked to sit outside the consultant's room whilst they both discussed my case.

When I was invited into the room I saw the consultant sitting behind his desk looking very pompous, which I'm sure was all an act in front of the junior doctor, for, when later I saw him alone, he dropped that silly facade and behaved normally. He turned out to be very nice.

"I've had a letter from the consultant of the hospital you attended," he said, adopting a superior manner. "He says that he thinks it is all emotional and I'm sure he is correct. He is very thorough." And he went on, "I want you to take these tablets. They are one of the tricyclics amitriptyline. There are also blue pills that go with them, but I don't want to confuse you with them at the moment. Take one capsule each night and after a week you will feel better in the mornings, and after the second week you will feel better in the afternoon, and in the third week...all gone." He lifted his hands in the air. It was just as if he was talking to a child, assuring it that all those nasty little things would soon go away. "I want you to take them at 9 o'clock each evening and you are not to miss one night...if you do, they won't work," he added.

I did as I was told and took the 75 mg amitriptyline capsule every evening.

To my great joy it did improve the condition of my stomach, but I was still plagued with constant loose stools.

A week after I had seen the psychiatrist, I saw again the consultant at the other South London hospital. But he showed no interest in me whatsoever. By handing the responsibility over to what he thought was the right department—psychiatric—he obviously felt he had done his duty.

I told him I was indeed brighter in myself and my stomach had improved, but when I still complained of constant diarrhoea he showed his impatience.

"Oh, you've got an irritable bowel," he snapped, and promptly handed me a leaflet on the subject and that was the end of that.

However, after only a fortnight on the prescribed drug amitriptyline my sickness returned and I again became very weepy. I had an appointment at St Thomas' Hospital a few days later, and on that occasion I saw a very young lady psychiatrist. She was a stand-in doctor.

I told her of my recurring problems but she didn't have the confidence to deal with it herself, so she rushed out of the room and went off to discuss what best to do with the consultant.

When she came back she said, "The consultant said you are to take two 75mg tablets of amitriptyline at night plus one blue pill in the morning."

After a couple of nights on that dosage the condition of my stomach improved once again, but as before, not the diarrhoea. I now had to contend with a new set of problems. I was obliged to keep drinking all day, my mouth was so dry I could barely speak and for the first couple of hours after getting up in the morning I found it difficult to move my arms and legs. It was as if I was paralysed and, farther more, I had unsightly red lumps all over my face and there was something else, something that I found very worrying indeed—I had a ringing sound in my head.

The consultant had not warned me of the possible side effects of the drug amitriptyline. In fact, some time later, when I saw him and told him that I found the side effects unacceptable, he evaded the issue. "Amitriptyline is a widely used and well tested drug. It's been on the market for 30 years," I was told.

I am sure that was the case but the drug did certainly have severe side effects, so why did he pretend they didn't exist?

The next time I went to the psychiatric clinic I saw yet another psychiatrist. This time it was a fair-haired lady in her forties. I thought she was a complete neurotic, but I got along with her very well, she did at least treat me as a responsible and intelligent adult, albeit with problems.

"My stomach has improved since I've been taking two 75mg tablets of amitriptyline, but I am still plagued by diarrhoea," I told her, which to my amazement, she dismissed out of hand and she wrote in her notes, diarrhoea improving, which I knew was absolute nonsense. "And I can't move my hands and legs properly in the mornings."

"Take them earlier in the evening," she advised. Then continued, "They will also give you a dry mouth and make you dream. Antidepressants are only effective when they make the mouth dry."

But as for the ringing in my head she had no answer, and when I pointed out the red blotches on my face, she looked concerned but made no comment.

She then went on at great length to explain that my stress was producing my psychological depression with symptoms which could affect my stomach, making me vomit and giving me diarrhoea and migraine. She said, "Your involuntary nervous system, because of the stress, pumps too much adrenaline into the stomach which acts on your vagus nerve causing all your problems. Amitriptyline acts on the vagus nerve stopping the excess adrenaline from doing harm, but if you do exercises such as walking and swimming you will use up all your adrenaline and also produce endorphins which are natural antidepressants. Amitriptyline and prottraden never produce dependence, but drugs such as diazepan, ativan and tranxene do." She then urged me to read a book called *Self-help for Nervous Suffering* by Dr Claire Weeks and made an appointment for me to see her in three weeks time.

I found the book in the local library, took it home and read it thoroughly. It was indeed very informative and I am sure very helpful for people with real nervous problems, but it didn't help me in the least.

However, by the time my appointment came a few weeks later, I had found the side effects of the drug amitriptyline so intolerable that I was determined to get off them at the earliest possible opportunity. I hated the rash on my face, the ringing in my head and the paralysis I felt in my limbs in the morning, even though I was taking them earlier in the evening as she had recommended. But she was completely dumbfounded when I told her of my intention to get off the drug, and after a long pause she said, "There's no other drug I could recommend. Amitriptyline is the best. The others would be useless. I'll drop them by half and give them to you in tablets of 25 mg so that it will be easier for me to get you off them." And after pondering for a moment she added, "I could give you prottraden, their side effects are not so severe."

She immediately wrote out a prescription and I promised to give them a try.

That evening, as instructed, I took the 75 mg capsule of prottraden but, alas, I woke up the following morning with an inexplicable pain all down my left arm. Nevertheless, I took them again the following night, but when I woke up again with the same pain I decided that that was the end of that drug.

That night I went back on the drug amitriptyline, but instead of taking 150 mg l only took 75mg, reducing the dosage by half.

After only a few days, however, back came the nausea and sickness. So, after all my persevering with the drug, I was back to square one. The drug was not curing my symptoms and knowing that taking 75 mg of the drug was useless I decided to get off the wretched drug once and for all, which I did in just three weeks, but I wasn't prepared for the consequences.

In fairness to the psychiatrists, nobody had recommended that I stopped taking the drug that quickly. It was, of course, a foolish thing to do. For three days after I had completely stopped taking the drug, as I was getting out of the bath in the morning I began to pant heavily, gasping for breath. My muscles went weak and I collapsed to the floor. I continued to gasp for breath for some time; I thought I was going to die. It was very frightening and I had never experienced anything like it before.

Eventually, the panting eased and I was able to get up and dress. But I still felt very ill.

That particular morning, I had a ticket for a dress rehearsal at Covent Garden, which I was determined not to miss—opera being one of my great passions. Thinking that my symptoms might pass, my husband drove me there in the car. They didn't, and no sooner had I entered the auditorium to take my seat than I once again felt my chest tighten up. My heart began to thump and I gasped for breath, falling to the ground. I kept trying to get up, only to collapse again.

I knew it was because I had stopped taking the very powerful drug too quickly. I should have taken a couple of months, not weeks, to get off it.

An attendant at the Opera House noticed my distress, informed my husband and sent for an ambulance. It arrived in four minutes. I was helped into the ambulance by my husband and one of the ambulance men and off we sped to the nearest hospital, which was St Thomas'. The ambulance men tried to liven up the atmosphere by trying to make a joke out of everything, but I wept profusely during the whole journey, and the attendant ambulance man had to keep propping me up in my seat because I kept collapsing to the floor. It was just as well it was St Thomas' Hospital because they had all my notes. But I sobbed, "Perhaps they won't see me."

"Oh, they'll see you if you are brought there in an ambulance," one of the ambulance men assured me.

I was wheeled into the waiting hall of the department called Scutari and was told by a nurse to wait until the doctor came to attend to me. It wasn't long before a young man came out of an adjoining room and, without glancing in my direction, walked briskly across the hall commanding as he went along, "Come into the room." It wasn't a good start.

My husband helped me out of the wheelchair and although I was very wobbly I managed to walk slowly into the room.

By the tine I reached the room the psychiatrist had seated himself at his desk. He had a very bored, arrogant, supercilious look on his face. I disliked him at once. As soon as I had seated myself he asked Irritably, "What's the problem?"

I went on at length to explain that I had been taking the drug amitriptyline, 150 mg a night, and that I had reduced the dosage to nil after only three weeks because I hated the side effects so much. I told him that I thought the panting, rapid beating of the heart and collapsing was the result of coming off the drug too soon.

He dismissed that out of hand and snapped, "You've had a panic attack."

"I've never had a panic attack in my life," I retorted. But he wasn't listening.

"With a panic attack that severe you'll have to take amitriptyline for at least another six months—full dose," he said. And seeing the look of horror on my face he exclaimed. "It's a wonderful drug!"

Well it might be for some people I thought, but it wasn't for me and I had no intention of taking it again. And becoming increasingly tired of his overbearing, obnoxious manner I began to show my contempt for him.

"I'm here to help you," he said gently, immediately altering his manner.

"Well it doesn't seem like it," I retorted.

He just glanced down.

"I refuse to have anything more to do with amitriptyline," I said.

"Very well," he said, "I'll give you another drug. It's called prottraden but you'll have to take the full dose."

I didn't bother to argue further but I didn't intend taking that drug either.

He quickly wrote out a prescription and handed it to me.

"I'd better examine you before you go," he said with a sigh, and he led me into another room where I was told to undress and lie on the bed.

He tested my arms and legs for any weakness and then said contemptuously, "There's nothing wrong with you," before walking smartly out of the room.

It had been such a horrible experience and a waste of time that I wished I hadn't needed to be taken there.

The following week I had an appointment to see the lady psychiatrist and I told her what had happened. "It was because I had reduced the dosage too quickly," I told her.

"You've had a panic attack," she said immediately.

"I don't have panic attacks," I replied. But she too wasn't listening.

"I've had panic attacks and so has my daughter," she went on excitedly, her face beginning to flush, which was something that wasn't hard to believe.

She quickly got up from her seat and almost running out of the room she said, "I must get a paper bag."

I sat there drinking the carton of coffee I had taken in with me awaiting her return. After about five minutes the door suddenly burst open and she stood there holding a paper bag. She excitedly began to demonstrate how to use it. "You're hyperventilating," she said, which didn't mean anything to me at the time. She went on, "Hyperventilating is over breathing. Your heart suddenly races and you feel short of breath and you keep panting, but in fact you are taking in more breath than you need and your limbs go weak and you collapse. By breathing into the paper bag you take in more carbon dioxide." She handed me the paper bag and I breathed into it as directed. "Now you know what to do when you have a panic attack again," she said, sighing with relief that she had imparted that bit of knowledge.

Since I had refused to have anything more to do with amitriptyline or prottraden she was at a loss as to what to prescribe.

"I'll write a letter to the psychologist and she will give you an appointment," she said at last.

Because I was still worried about the red stains on my face she said, "I'll make an appointment for you to see Skins," and, once again, she rushed out of the room.

The department was at the other end of the psychiatric department and she soon returned saying, 'They'll give you an appointment in three weeks' time," and it was left at that.

As soon as I had left off the drug the ringing in my head stopped and the lumps on my face disappeared, but I was left with all my usual symptoms.

The psychiatrists, no doubt, believed they were doing the right thing in prescribing the drug to help my emotional state and ease my sickness, but what they were doing was merely masking the real cause of my devastating illness.

To help me get over what I put down to be the withdrawal effects of the drug, I went to my GP. My body felt like an electric wire. I couldn't sit still. I told her what had happened and she gave me chlorapromazine tablets. She told me to take them three times a day, which was ludicrous. I took one in the morning and couldn't keep awake for the rest of the day, so I didn't take any more.

As for my appointment with Skins, I saw a young dark-haired specialist who said, matter-of-factly, "The broken red veins are permanent and the red stains will fade in time, but we are talking about three to four months." He gave me a cortisone ointment to rub in every night.

Although the lumps had gone, the red stains had remained and they took considerably longer than a few months to fade, but they did fade and for the broken veins some time later I went along to the Delia Collins beauty salon in Knightsbridge, and the lady who runs the salon, Delia Collins' daughter, did a very good job in removing them—for which I was eternally grateful.

Incidentally, it appears that the specialists had never heard of anyone else suffering a rash or red blotches on their face after using the drug amitriptyline—or so they said.

The psychologist proved no help whatsoever, as I had expected. She spent considerable time in taking down a lot of details, but then just handed me a tape saying, "It's a relaxation tape. Listen to it every day and try to relax."

Unfortunately, I needed more than just relaxing to help solve my problems.

CHAPTER 4

Around the same time I had been given the name of two spiritual healers.

They lived in Reigate and their names were Irene and Gerald Sowter. People travelled great distances to be given spiritual healing and spirit operations which Irene gave. Their successes were always being written about in the Psychic News.

Reigate is quite a distance from where I live, but I managed to drive myself there in the car. I had to make an appointment well in advance because they were always so booked up. They healed on Tuesday and Thursday afternoons and their Healing Centre was in the basement of their large house.

I waited in the fairly large waiting room along with the many other people who came for healing. At the other end of the room there was a small chapel and the room was filled with beautiful soft music. It had a very peaceful and calming effect.

When it was my turn, Irene Sowter led me through a small door into the healing room, where there were a number of beds partitioned off by curtains. It all ran very smoothly.

I lay on one of the beds and Irene laid her hands on me. She asked me what was my particular problem and I told her everything I was experiencing.

Unfortunately she didn't appear to take me very seriously because she dismissed it by saying, "All I'm getting from the spirits is, 'tell her to leave off the chips'," which didn't go down very well with me, as you can imagine, because I really was feeling very ill. Needless to say, I didn't go again but she did give me a spirit operation a year or two later.

Because the psychiatrists had failed so miserably to improve my physical condition I felt I should go back to the Gastrointestinal clinic at

St Thomas' Hospital, so I made an appointment and stressed that I would like to see the consultant.

By that time, I was in the most deplorable state. I had diarrhoea and sickness almost every day, even pain in my stomach. My muscles ached all over my body and I had frequent sores on the sides of my mouth. I had a succession of throat infections for which I was obliged to take even more antibiotics. My body and my mind seemed to be giving way in all directions.

The consultant was a very polite and considerate man and I liked him, but he had no answer to my problems. I did, however, tell him that a polyp was found after a bowel x-ray in 1976 and he said, "I'll arrange a colonoscopy for you right away. It will be in three weeks time. The polyp will be taken away."

The man at the reception desk told me that the waiting list for a colonoscopy at the hospital was three months, but because it was the consultant who wanted it I could have the colonoscopy in about three weeks time.

Meanwhile, for my persistent diarrhoea he gave me codeine tablets, but when I took them as prescribed it stopped me from going to the toilet altogether, so I only took them now and again.

A few days after I had seen the consultant I heard from the hospital that my colonoscopy had been arranged for the middle of August 1985.

I thought I would try alternative medicine in the meantime and I telephoned Neal's Yard and made an appointment to see a homeopath. He spent a considerable amount of time asking a lot of questions and then gave me pulsutilla for constitutional purposes, saying it would give me a feeling of well-being, which alas it didn't, and when I saw him again and told him that I was still suffering all the same symptoms he replied, "If you are worried about anything go and see your doctor," which I didn't regard as being very helpful.

I then saw an advertisement in a health magazine for a holistic clinic. I rang the clinic and spoke to a lady. Referring to her husband she said,

"He can tell what is wrong with you by looking into your eyes. It's called Iridology." And she went on, "Then we will give you homeopathic treatment. You will also receive healing. We are both healers. My father is a doctor and at first he refused to have anything to do with homeopathy, but now even he is converted after seeing what we achieve."

I thought their fee was a bit steep but I was so desperate for help I would have paid almost anything at that moment in time and I didn't hesitate to make an appointment for a few days later.

They lived in a block of flats overlooking the Thames and I don't know how I reached there that morning. I was obliged to go by public transport. I had had severe diarrhoea earlier in the morning and my body ached all over. I also felt slightly disorientated.

There was an entry-phone at the entrance to the flat and I rang their number. A female voice answered, "My husband will meet you downstairs and escort you up to the flat," she said.

A short, stocky, dark-haired man opened the door and he led me upstairs to the first floor flat, which was very small but tastefully furnished. A very pleasant lady greeted me and she looked and spoke very middle class.

"Would you like a cup of herbal tea?" she asked sweetly.

I accepted gratefully and she went off into the kitchen while I made myself comfortable in the sitting room. Her husband had disappeared into another room. When she came back with the tea she sat down and began chatting away to me. She seemed surprised at the way I behaved saying, "The people who come here are always very confused."

I made no comment.

Her husband came back into the room bringing with him a large drawing of an iris. He then proceeded to look first into my right eye and then the left, marking everything he saw on to the drawing of the iris. It took a long time. His wife meanwhile busied herself elsewhere, coming into the room every now and then to enquire how he was getting on.

When he had at last finished she studied the markings on the iris and then said, "All your organs are in place…you should be very grateful. We had one woman who couldn't breathe properly because her whole inside was enlarged and not in position, causing her breathing problems." I sat listening carefully to all she had to say and she went on, "One mother brought her daughter to us. She was suffering from severe depression and she was overjoyed when we told her that the problem was physical." She didn't elaborate on the issue and continued, "Another woman passed a kidney stone after we had given her healing. She went straight into the toilet and passed it.

I told her of all my distressing symptoms and the fact that I was going into hospital in a few weeks to have a polyp removed from my bowel.

"We can get rid of polyps for you," she said confidently. "We had one woman who had a polyp in her nose."

"And it disappeared?" I asked incredulously.

"Yes," she replied. "But if you prefer to have surgery that's up to you."

I had no intention of giving up my colonoscopy so I declined the offer.

"You've got a lesion in your bowel," her husband said. "It shows up. But they'll find that."

"Will it help my diarrhoea?" I asked hopefully.

"Yes," he replied. "But it won't do anything for your stomach."

After sorting out some homeopathic remedies the lady said, "If I had a fair-haired daughter I would definitely give her pulsutilla. It's for constitutional purposes."

She also gave me some Bach Flower remedies, which included the famous Rescue remedy which is said to be excellent for shock. "I am never without it. I carry it in my handbag everywhere," she said. "I'll also give you some bowel powder. It's made especially by a lady. I'll give you her address, then if you want some more you can send for it yourself. You put the powder in capsules."

She went off to look for some capsules but she couldn't find any. She was pleased, however, when I told her I had some at home. I had bought them to make ginger root capsules because I had read that they were far more effective than the seasickness drugs which are on the market and furthermore they don't make you sleepy. I have used them on a number of occasions since and found them invaluable.

"I'm going to throw everything at you," she said, probably guessing that she wouldn't be seeing me again.

Once again she hurried out of the room, returning clasping what looked like a hot water bottle. But it turned out to be a rectal douche.

"You fill it full of water and the tube coming from it you insert into the rectum. It will clean out your bowels," she said, as she turned to demonstrate how it worked, looking very funny in the process. And she went on to say, "A lady I know says you are not clean inside unless you go to the toilet three times a day. I only go once so I'm not clean," she laughed.

I didn't say anything but it seemed a bit of an exaggeration on the lady's part.

"Now we will give you some healing," she said.

"Have you ever had spiritual healing before?"

"Yes," I replied. "I go to the SAGB on a Sunday whenever I can."

She seemed pleased. It was true, I had first started going there when my eyes were bad and I had continued to go.

I was asked to sit on an upright chair and they both put their hands on me. After about fifteen minutes she asked, "Are you feeling any different?"

Sadly, I was not feeling in the least bit different but I gave a non-committal answer, not wanting to disappoint them. I paid them and left. I had been at the flat for two and a half hours.

I took the pulsutilla and the Bach Flower remedies, but the bowel tonic only aggravated my already deplorable condition and I didn't take any more.

A fortnight before my colonoscopy I had such severe pains in my stomach that I telephoned my GP. Since I had told her about my ambulance trip to St Thomas' Hospital she hadn't failed to visit me. But she didn't bother to hide her feelings.

"It's all in the head," she snapped with frustration. "Would you like a psychiatrist to visit you today?"

Why not? I thought, so I simply nodded.

"If you want a home visit you'll have to see a psychiatrist from another hospital," she said.

"That's perfectly all right," I replied.

"The consultant will call today," she assured. She then proceeded to telephone the nearest psychiatric hospital, telling them that it was an emergency.

I waited all day to no avail. When the consultant did turn up it was a week later. So much for the emergency, I thought.

He was a short, Asian-looking gentleman in his late fifties or early sixties. He sat on the settee and took out a scrap of paper on which he scribbled all my answers to his questions.

"Why did you stop going to St Thomas' Hospital?" he asked. It was a fact that didn't seem to please him.

"Because all they had to offer was amitriptyline and I couldn't take the side effects any longer," I answered.

"Not many people can," he replied.

"I've gone back to taking surmontil," I told him. I had been given some by my GP at some time or another in the past.

"It's an excellent antidepressant," he said.

"It certainly doesn't have the side effects that amitriptyline has," I replied.

Knowing that I was going into hospital to have a polyp removed in a week's time he said, "But I can't do anything for you now. I don't want to confuse you. Let's see what the result of the operation will be first. Contact me when it's over with." And it was left at that.

But I failed to see what a significant difference the removal of a polyp would make to my condition. And I was right, it didn't make the slightest difference!

CHAPTER 5

The day for me to enter hospital arrived. It was on a Monday in August and it was a beautiful day. After packing the necessaries into a suitcase I called a minicab which took me to the hospital. My husband was on tour in Greece at the time but he was returning the following day.

On arriving at the hospital I reported to the reception desk and was told to go to a certain ward. I climbed the stairs to the ward and then introduced myself to the sister who led me to my bed. It was in a room with three other patients. The ward, incidentally, had a spectacular view overlooking the Thames, especially at night when all the lights were lit.

Two of the patients in the room had had strokes and were paralysed down one side. They had been admitted to hospital because their blood pressure had risen dangerously high. One was a black lady who only looked in her forties. The other lady was in her sixties. I felt very sorry for them both. The black lady seemed to take it all in her stride while the other lady said, "I only live from day to day now."

The third lady had pains in her stomach and was in hospital for tests.

I didn't undress because I didn't want to lie in bed all day, and when the consultant arrived on his morning rounds I sat on the bed to answer his questions. He had with him the friendly doctor I had seen at the clinic and none other than the Australian doctor who did nothing but bellow at everyone. My heart sank when I saw him and he turned out to be the doctor on ward duty during the whole of my stay there.

I began telling the consultant and his retinue of doctors about my whole array of symptoms. They listened politely but the consultant didn't comment when I had finished. I was clearly only there for the removal of the polyp.

"Who's going to carry out the operation?" the consultant asked and the nice friendly doctor put up his hand. "Do your best and see what you can find," he said to him. The consultant then continued on his rounds.

Not long afterwards, the young Australian doctor came rushing up to me and he said pointedly, "You'll be having your operation tomorrow. That's the only reason you're here."

But I didn't need to be told that, it had been made obvious and I didn't bother to mention all my debilitating symptoms for the rest of my stay there.

The Australian doctor then said, with some irritation, "They usually come in on Sunday. Now we'll have to work quickly."

He went charging off and soon afterwards the sister came up with a tumbler full of very chalky liquid which I was required to swallow.

"Drink plenty of water," she said. "You must drink at least three jarfuls today."

"I can't drink water," I replied with a grimace.

"Well, we'll put some orange squash in it," she said.

Soon afterwards, and for the rest of the day and night, I was obliged to run to the toilet. I didn't sleep all night.

The following morning I was prepared for my operation and the doctor again came rushing up to me.

"I'm sorry, but you won't be having your operation today, it's been delayed until Wednesday," he said. "We'll give you some more liquid."

"Oh, not more," I protested.

"Yes," he said, "but we'll give it to you early so that you can have a night's rest." And he added with glee, "You'll have the cleanest bowel yet."

I was given more chalky liquid and the process began again. But in the afternoon the sister allowed me out of hospital to walk on the embankment with my husband. It was another warm, sunny day.

That night I did have a more restful time but I hardly slept because one of the ladies snored heavily the whole night.

In the morning I bathed and at about 10 a.m. the nurse came and gave me a gown to put on. Soon afterwards my bed, with me in it, was taken downstairs by the lift and wheeled into the operating room. I saw the nice doctor who gave me an injection. I felt drowsy immediately but I remember waking up and saying to him, "Don't forget the polyps….Don't forget the polyps." He just smiled at me.

After I was taken back to the ward I slept for an hour or two, but as soon as I woke up the young Australian doctor came rushing up to my bed and he said excitedly, "It's good news. The lump was taken straight to the lab and analysed. There's no cancer."

Of course it was good news, but I wasn't in the least elated by it and he looked disappointed. I knew I still had to contend with all my physical problems and that was a sobering thought and I told him so. He didn't answer. It wasn't, after all, the reason why I was in hospital. "We'll see you again in six months' time," he said before leaving my bed. "You'll have another colonoscopy." The doctor was really not too bad. He just had an unfortunate manner.

The following week I toured Denmark, Norway and Sweden. But, as to be expected it turned out to be a bit of a disaster. My condition had deteriorated considerably since I had visited America the year before. No longer did maxolon tablets help my stomach. My tongue would go dry and I had a horrible feeling in my stomach, sometimes accompanied by pain. On one or two occasions I thought I would have to fly home.

I had obtained Marie Treben's book called *Health from God's Pharmacy* and in it she recommends a herbal mixture called 'Swedish Bitters' for a great many complaints, and passing through Germany I managed to buy some. Because it contained alcohol it could not be imported from Germany and Baldwins, the famous herbalist, at that time, had to sell it in powder form. But you could make the mixture yourself by first adding 1½ litres of whisky or gin and leaving it to stand by a stove for fourteen days. The herbs, however, didn't help my condition in the least.

After arriving back in England I immediately contacted the consultant psychiatrist, just as I had been told to do. However, he didn't get around to seeing me for many weeks after that, although his clinic was only a hundred yards away from my home and was far from busy, as I later found out.

Meanwhile, still desperate to find help, I saw an advertisement in the local press for a hypnotist and telephoned to make an appointment. One was arranged for the following week.

He lived in a detached house in Kent. My husband drove me there and waited in the car whilst I went into the house for treatment.

He was running late, so I was obliged to wait for three quarters of an hour. I sat in a room with three old ladies who, at first, I thought were patients, but it turned out that they lived there. The hypnotist's wife looked after them. Press cuttings of his achievements were pinned to a board and I read them carefully. He seemed to have had considerable success.

When I saw him for the first time I had a bit of a shock for he was an unusual looking man. He had a large square face and he sported a ginger beard which emphasized the squareness. He had a deep sonorous voice, in fact, the deepest I have ever heard. It was no wonder he was a hypnotist. His deep voice would send anyone to sleep. He asked me all that was troubling me and I told him everything I could—my whole catalogue of symptoms, especially my red, dry tongue and horrible feelings in my stomach.

"Sit comfortably in the chair," he said slowly. "Close your eyes and just listen to my voice." It wasn't difficult to do that. "I will count slowly up to ten and by that time you will be totally relaxed," he said. He counted to ten and then went on, "I am the only person who can hypnotise you. You will respond only to my voice." I listened intently to everything he said. "Now I am going to count up to five and clap my hands. After that you will open your eyes and be totally awake," he said.

He counted slowly up to five and then clapped his hands so loudly I nearly jumped out of my seat.

He repeated the process about five times and then said, "You will be ready to be hypnotised when I see you again," which was disappointing since I was hoping to be given healing suggestions right away.

I had told him that I was taking the drug surmontil and he gave me some leaflets on the dangers of taking tranquillizers saying, somewhat aghast, "We must get you off them as soon as possible."

He stressed the necessity of regular treatment and I made an appointment for the following week.

I hadn't been put to sleep but I knew that you only needed to be very relaxed for his words to penetrate into the subconscious. I had read Emil Coue's book called 'Auto Suggestion' and had tried repeating, "Every day and in every way I am getting better and better," twenty times before I went to sleep. He tells us that a general suggestion is more successful than a more detailed one. However, nothing seemed to help me.

When next I saw the hypnotist I sat in the chair and did my best to relax. He counted up to ten in his deep voice and then said, "Imagine a door that is fully open out of which all your cares and worries are being swept with a broom. When the door is finally closed that will be the end of all your troubles. The red tongue and all the horrible feelings you have in your stomach will stop. Now imagine yourself going up a hill and when you reach the top that will be the end of your pathetic condition. I am now closing the door a quarter and you are beginning to climb the hill."

He repeated the suggestions a number of times and then slowly counted up to five and clapped his hands. He then began questioning me at length, noting my answers.

"Did you see a door?" he asked.

"Yes, I did vaguely," I replied.

"Did you see a hill?" he then asked.

I nodded and on it went until he finally asked, "Do you feel better?"

I didn't, but I gave my usual non-committal answer.

I made appointments for the following couple of weeks, hoping for the best. At each session he continued to give me the suggestions that the door was closing more and more and that I was getting farther and farther up the hill and my troubles were getting less and less and I was getting better and better and so on. And then at the end of about the fourth session he told me that he was going on a lecture tour on the continent for a few weeks. I was a bit put out because he had stressed the importance of not interrupting the sessions.

"It can't be helped," he said brusquely when I reminded him of it.

However, by that time I had received the long awaited appointment to see the consultant psychiatrist. The appointment was for 10 a.m. and the waiting room was empty apart from a young girl. She was called into his consulting room first and after about twenty minutes she re-emerged sobbing her heart out. She hadn't been sobbing when she went in and the consultant, looking distinctly embarrassed, tried to comfort her. It didn't look very promising.

When it was my turn I went into his consulting room and just sat and waited for him to speak.

"The trouble with you is that you don't listen to what you're told," he said impatiently.

I don't know where he had got that from but I didn't argue with him.

"Since you don't want to take amitriptyline any longer we'll try bolvidon," he said and then he added, "but you must do as I say." I nodded my agreement.

He wrote out a prescription for bolvidon and told me to make an appointment with the receptionist for four week's time. I took the drug that night, just as he had prescribed, but alas, the following morning I got out of bed and immediately fell to the floor. I was that giddy. And when I did manage to get up I was groping all over the place and for the rest of the day I actually felt as if I was going mad.

"If that's what bolvidon does to me then that's the end of that drug," I said to myself and I didn't take any more. Instead I went back on the drug surmontil. Fortunately I still had some left.

Because the drug had had such a devastating effect on me I thought I should see the consultant psychiatrist again, so I telephoned and asked if I could see him earlier than my appointed time in four weeks.

His secretary answered and said, "The consultant is away on holiday for a few weeks but you can see his stand-in if you want to."

I agreed to do that.

The young doctor I saw the following week turned out to be very polite, sympathetic and sensible. He stood up when I entered the consulting room, shook my hand and introduced himself. I wasn't used to that kind of treatment. "I'm here for a few weeks while the consultant is on holiday," he said.

I sat down and immediately poured out all my troubles. He listened carefully and noted down all I said, after which he said, "Since you don't want to take bolvidon or amitriptyline I'll put you on surmontil."

"I'm already taking 50mg a night," I told him.

"But that's only a beginner's dosage," he said. "We must raise that to 100mg a night. We have to get your nerves right."

I still had my appointment with the consultant in three week's time and I intended keeping it. But my mind and body continued on its downward spiral and I now began to have what I thought to be panic attacks. My chest would tighten and I would begin gasping for breath and because I had taken in too much oxygen my muscles would weaken and I would fall to the ground.

One Sunday I kept panting all day, I just couldn't get my breath. My chest felt so tight and I kept falling to the floor. But since it was Sunday we were obliged to call an emergency doctor and he came to the house very quickly. Emergency doctors never fail to visit you.

He examined me and then said, "Your thyroid gland could be causing the problem," and he wrote out a letter to give to my GP the following morning.

I made an appointment to see the GP and when she read the letter she seemed pleased. "A fresh opinion," she said with optimism.

I was sent to a South London hospital for a blood test. But, after a few days, because I was in such distress with my sickness and perpetual diarrhoea, I went to see her again and this time my husband came with me.

"You haven't got thyroid trouble," she said with a deep sigh. She had received the results of the blood test. Then, turning to my husband she said, "I don't know what is wrong with your wife. We give imodiurn for diarrhoea and maxolon for sickness but it doesn't seem to do any good."

No one seemed able to help me. However, in an attempt to stop the sickness I even went back on the drug amitriptyline. It had helped in the past but this time they made me so dizzy I couldn't walk about so I abandoned that idea.

I was now in total despair, not knowing what to do or where to turn, and so in desperation I asked the secretary of the consultant psychiatrist if I could see him a week earlier than my appointed time.

"Yes, he'll see you," she answered.

I waited patiently whilst he saw the same young lady. She was the only patient I ever saw there and as usual she came out of his room in tears.

When it was my turn I went into his room and sat opposite him at his desk. He looked up and glared at me.

"Let me tell you first of all that we can't keep on seeing you like this. You came the other week," he snapped.

"But if things go wrong," I attempted to say, but he completely ignored me and began furiously to turn over the pages of notes the young doctor had left for him. His face was purple with rage and he laughed scornfully as he turned over the pages. He simply could not contain his anger. And it was all because I had refused to take the wretched bolvidon tablets-the drug he had prescribed for me. My heart was beating so fast I felt I was going to collapse. This man was supposed to be treating me for my nerves and yet he showed no concern whatsoever at the effect his preposterous behaviour was having on me. I decided that I wasn't going to take any more and I got up and walked to the door saying, "Well if you don't want to see me...."

"Sit down, sit down," he said gently, somewhat surprised at my reaction to his appalling behaviour. Perhaps because he was so used to dealing with very disturbed patients he thought I couldn't fully comprehend what was going on and could be easily pacified. Of course, he was mistaken.

Nevertheless, I did sit down again thinking that he may now have regained his composure, but I was wrong because no sooner had I sat down again he leaned over his desk and glared at me. His face was totally contorted with rage and he said through clenched teeth, "This is the second time you've been here."

I couldn't believe what I was witnessing. There was I in desperate need of help and I had a consultant psychiatrist whose behaviour was that of a madman!

This time I didn't hesitate, I walked quickly to the door. I wanted to get out of the room as fast as I could. The man was totally irresponsible.

"Good-bye," I said in disgust.

But before leaving the room I quickly glanced back at him to find out his reaction to my walking out on him. He was just staring in front of him, totally stunned.

"Good-bye," he said chokingly.

Did he really think that I was so far removed from reality that I wouldn't react that way to his outrageous behaviour? God only knows. But what I did know was the devastating effect it had on me, for I walked home in a complete daze, shaking violently and it took me several hours to calm down. And, as with the other consultant, his behaviour could have had serious consequences.

My husband wanted to confront the psychiatrist but I stopped him. I saw no point. And even if I had written to the authorities about his behaviour, it was my word against his and I was merely his psychiatric patient—not a very good recommendation, so I didn't entertain the idea for long. He could have got away with murder. A year or two later, however, I was to encounter him again.

Alas, I didn't fare much better with the hypnotist. I went to see him again after he returned from his continental tour. He continued to give me the same suggestions, but although the door was almost closed and all my troubles should, supposedly, have been swept away and I was nearly at the top of the hill, I was in no way any better and I felt I had to be truthful with him.

"Well if you don't listen to what I'm saying," he replied sharply.

"But I do listen," I argued.

"You can't be listening," he replied, sounding even angrier. He began rummaging through the drawers of his desk and he took out some photographs. He held one up. "Look," he said, "this boy had psoriasis and he was cured." I didn't dispute the fact and he held up another photograph. "This man had a terrible pain in his shoulder. He couldn't work for years. It was psychosomatic and I cured him," he said and he added, sneeringly, "I have cured people who were in a much worse state than you."

"But what if it isn't psychosomatic but an infection throughout the body, there's nothing you can do about that," I replied, trying to be fair but he took no notice of what I said, he was too angry. He clearly had no time for his failures.

Finally, however, he said, "Since it is a lot of money and I can't do anything for you, I suggest you don't come again."

I left without making another appointment. But I meant what I said about my having an infection throughout the body. I had been thinking about that possibility for some time. But what infection? It was obviously something that the medical profession didn't recognise or seem to know anything about.

CHAPTER 6

I continued to go to the SAGB in Belgrave Square for healing. I went on a Sunday whenever I could manage it. Marjorie was my usual healer.

Several times I had asked to be put on the waiting list to see the famous healer Tom Johannson but they always refused. Although he healed on a Saturday morning when he was in London they kept telling me there simply was no point. I could never understand why, since I was prepared to wait months if necessary.

Around that time I saw an advert for a diagnostic healer in the Psychic News. I decided to contact her, thinking that she may be able to tell me what was wrong with me. She lived somewhere in the Midlands but she said, "I'm coming to London on a Sunday in a few week's time. Would you like me to visit you?"

I was delighted.

"I'm clairvoyant and clairaudient. I can hear spirit voices when I'm healing," she said, "and I have a number of patients to visit in London. I can easily fit you in.

"How much do you charge?" I asked.

"I only charge for expenses," she replied. "It's £20." I thought it a bit steep but I accepted it.

"I'll phone you to let you know which Sunday I'm coming to London," she said, and we left it at that.

Two weeks passed and she telephoned me. "I'm coming to London this Sunday," she said. "Is it all right to visit you at 2 p.m.?"

"Yes that will be fine," I replied.

I waited eagerly for Sunday to come and when it did the healer arrived at the house on time. I opened the door to see a smart looking lady in her forties. She had short red hair.

As she entered the house she said, "My husband is waiting in the car outside. I have one more patient to visit."

We sat down and I told her briefly the history of my ill health, after which she set about giving me healing. I sat on an upright chair and she stood behind me, placing her hands on my shoulders. Soon she was swaying back and forth and this went on for a quarter of an hour.

When she had finished she asked, "Did you feel anything?"

Alas I hadn't but I didn't say so, not wanting to discourage her.

"When I sway back and forth I know a lot of energy is going out of me," she said.

"What did the spirits say?" I asked eagerly, hoping for some reassurance that all would be well.

She sat on the settee and replied, "They said you could be a new person in six weeks," and then added quickly, "but that doesn't mean you will be…. but you could be."

I thought it a bit optimistic since I had been ill for so long and still didn't know what was wrong with me. However, she went on, "I can see a dark tunnel which you are now in, but at the end of the tunnel, I cannot only see light but sunlight." I found it encouraging. The medium from the SAGB had said something similar.

I then asked her to tell me of her successes and she said, "I had one lady who had taken valium for years and she found it hard to get off them. She shook from head to foot at first but we got her off them in four weeks. But then she was able to come to the clinic regularly. I had another woman who had a very painful back. She had x-rays and treatment but nothing relieved her. The spirits told me what to do and I maneuvered her spine back into position. It was something the doctors had missed. I still have letters from people thanking me for helping them."

I gave her a cheque for £20 and she left—promising to contact me when next she was in London.

She visited me on several occasions, telling me on one occasion, "The spirits say that you are a very talented lady and you haven't anywhere near finished using your talent."

Alas, when I couldn't detect any improvement in my seemingly hopeless condition I stopped seeing her, although I continued to go to the SAGB for healing.

One Sunday I went along there only to find that Marjorie had been taken ill with a heart condition, so I was obliged to see another healer. She was a very old lady with a deeply lined face but she was full of exuberance and spirit.

As soon as I lay on the bed in readiness to be healed I began to cry uncontrollably. She caressed my face with her hands whilst I poured out all my sorrows.

"I've been ill for years," I sobbed, "and nobody knows what's wrong with me, nobody helps me and I'm in total despair. I'm so depressed."

"I'd be depressed if I had been ill for years," she replied sympathetically in an effort to comfort me. "Let me see your tongue. That's what the doctor says, doesn't he? I'm a qualified nurse and I used to work in a hospital…years ago that is."

I held out my tongue.

"It's filthy," she screamed immediately. "Now you must brush it every day with a toothbrush, using salt water, or buy a gargle from the chemists. I always brush mine with a toothbrush. Look!" She held out a very healthy looking tongue and I promised to do as she had instructed.

I tried to relax as best I could on the bed and she held her hands over me for some time. When she had finished she exclaimed, "Look at your face! Look how relaxed it is!" And she led me to the cloakroom and insisted that I looked into the mirror.

"Look at it!" she repeated, almost jumping up with glee. And she added with conviction, "It's because you have had healing." However, all I could see were my red swollen eyes from crying. I was indeed a pitiful sight.

I thanked her for the healing and promised faithfully to see her again the following week.

The first thing I did the next morning was to go to a chemist shop and buy an antibacterial gargle. The chemist gave me Corsodyl saying, "That's what the dentists recommend."

I began gargling with it immediately and in a few day's time I noticed an improvement in my stomach condition. The red dry tongue had gone along with the pain in my stomach. All my other symptoms remained, but it was enough to convince me still further that I was suffering from some sort of infection throughout my body.

I was able to tell the healer that there had been some sort of improvement in my condition when next I saw her and after giving me healing she spent some time advising me what vitamin supplements to take. "I always take selenium," she said, "it helps my immune system."

However, after a week or so of gargling with Corsodyl I decided to make an appointment to see my GP yet again. I wanted to tell her I was convinced that my condition was due to an infection in the body.

She wasn't pleased to see me and showed her irritation when I said, "I've been gargling with Corsodyl and my condition has improved so I've clearly got some sort of infection in the mouth."

"I've never heard of Corsodyl," she sighed.

"It's for infections in the mouth," I told her and I then went on to ask if I could have more of the drug nystatin. "I still have sores at the corners of my mouth and frequent throat infections. I'm convinced my condition is because of an infection throughout the body." I was almost pleading with her.

She gave another deep sigh. "Let me look at your tongue," she said irritably. I held out my tongue. "You definitely haven't got thrush so you don't need nystatin!"

My heart began to pound and I began to panic when I could see that she was going to refuse to prescribe the drug which I thought was my salvation.

However, I was determined not to leave the surgery without a prescription and I demanded, "I want nystatin tablets and nystatin cream."

Very well," she conceded, "I'll give you ten day's supply of nystatin tablets and the cream." But she did it just to get rid of me and not because she thought it would do me any good.

After taking the course of tablets I was no better, and so I decided to try another approach. The nystatin I had been prescribed was woefully inadequate, but I didn't know that at the time. I went back to the surgery and asked the receptionist to find out from the doctor if it was possible to have antibiotics for the infection I felt I had in the bowel. That's how ignorant I was concerning my illness.

Back she came with the message, "The doctor says antibiotics do not work on the bowel and that no drug would kill the germs there."

Determined not to give up I telephoned a chemist and asked if there were any drugs that cleared up infections in the bowel.

"Yes," he replied and he gave me the name of a brand which I wrote down. I was excited.

I went again to the surgery and asked the receptionist if I could see the doctor. The surgery was nearly empty. I showed her the name of the drug I had written down and said, "I would like some of these tablets."

"I'll see what the doctor has to say about it" she replied and she telephoned through to the doctor and told her of my request.

When she put down the telephone she said, "I'm afraid the doctor says she's never heard of the tablets."

Immediately something in my brain snapped and I became hysterical. "I knew she wouldn't, I knew she wouldn't," I shouted. "The chemist told me about them. Tell her to telephone the chemist."

"Will you stop shouting," the receptionist said, but I was unable to control myself. I was frantic that she was denying me my only hope of recovery.

"Tell her to telephone them right now," I kept insisting. The telephone rang and the receptionist answered it.

"It's Mrs Barrett," she said and after a minute or two she replaced the receiver. Looking up at me she said, "It was the doctor. She asked who was shouting in the waiting room and when I told her she said that you'll have to find another doctor, she can't have shouting in the surgery."

It was all I needed. I was in total despair and I felt as though I was going to collapse on the spot.

"And where do I find one?" I managed to mumble.

"Oh, there's plenty around," the receptionist replied, nonchalantly.

The patient in the waiting room gave me a sympathetic look as I passed her on my way out of the surgery.

My husband collected the medical cards as soon as possible and transferred them to a clinic not far from home. He encountered the doctor on his way out of the surgery.

"You have left me with a very sick woman," he told her, but she had just smiled her usual sickly smile. I had never liked her. I knew that under her facade of gentleness there was a bitter, nasty woman. The facade had dropped on a few occasions. She did have a club foot; perhaps that was the reason for her bitterness.

The clinic comprised of two middle-aged men and an elderly lady. Immediately I made an appointment to see one of the male doctors. I told him of all my symptoms; the sickness, the diarrhoea, my general malaise and my so-called panic attacks.

"I'll give you maxalon, that will cure your sickness," he said confidently.

"Are you sure?" I asked, knowing very well that it wouldn't cure it. It would merely stop me from feeling sick.

"Absolutely," he replied. And then he added smugly, "But I know what's wrong with you, it's all on your face…anxiety. You must get rid of your anxiety. I suggest you see a psychiatrist and go to management and relaxation classes."

I nodded. There was after all nothing to lose. The following week I had an appointment to see a lady who I thought was a psychiatrist, but she turned out to be a psychiatric nurse. She took down all the necessary details in a very half-soaked manner but I burst into tears during the interview. She gave me a tissue and said, "You are far too beautiful and intelligent to be left on the scrap heap!"

I was determined not to be left on the scrap heap if I could possibly help it. If only I knew what was wrong with me.

"The management and relaxation classes will begin after Christmas and I'll write and give you the details later on," she said before I left.

They didn't in fact start until the end of February. Meanwhile I continued to see my healer at the SAGB. She knew that cleaning my tongue had not been the answer to my continued ill-health and when next I saw her she said, "I've been meditating about you. It's something that is affecting your whole body." And she went on, "I have an acquaintance, through my healing. He is an osteopath and he runs an allergy clinic in North London and at Harley Street. I told him all about you. I told him about your tongue and he said without any hesitation, 'I know what's wrong with her'. He's a very young man but extremely friendly." She seemed excited about it. "Ring me on Wednesday after 8 p.m. and I will give you all the details," she ended by saying.

When Wednesday arrived I telephoned her and, true to her word, she gave me all the details of the young man in question. His allergy clinic was quite a distance away in North London and she kindly offered to take me there, but I told her I would be able to manage it alone. Since she was old I didn't want to overburden her. Immediately after I had telephoned her I rang the clinic, hoping that I would be lucky enough to catch him there. I did.

"I was just about to leave the clinic," he said, somewhat out of breath. I told him that a lady healer, an acquaintance of his had recommended that I saw him.

"Oh yes, I remember her," he replied.

"Could I make an appointment to see you at your Harley Street clinic because it's much nearer for me?" I asked.

"I would prefer you to come to my North London clinic. The fee is much less and I will be able to give you more time," he replied.

I didn't argue. I made an appointment to see him one morning the following week. I had been ill for two years and was in the most lamentable state. I had practically given up all hope of regaining my health and it was in that sad plight that I set off to see the osteopath a week later.

As I had expected, it turned out to be a very long journey. I travelled most of the way by tube and all the rest of the way by bus, alighting right outside his clinic. I couldn't fail to miss it, there was a large notice board outside.

I was told by the lady receptionist that I would have to wait about three quarters of an hour before being seen. There were two ladies waiting in the tiny waiting room. Both had back problems so, to while away the time, I went to a cafe just opposite the clinic and had a cup of coffee.

I returned just in time to be ushered upstairs to see the osteopath.

He was, indeed, very young and boyish looking, brimming over with health and vitality. I envied him.

"Sit down," he said, pointing to a chair that was shaped like an 'S'. "I designed that myself. A pianist friend of mine is very interested in it. It stops backache." I didn't dispute it, but I kept slipping off it.

"What can I do for you?" he asked, smiling broadly at me.

Immediately I poured out all my troubles to him. "I have nausea, vomiting and diarrhoea. I keep getting sores on the corners of my mouth and I have frequent throat infections. My chest feels very tight and I pant and fall to the ground. I have a distant feeling, terrible depression and my nerves are in the most atrocious state."

Without any hesitation he said, "I only have to spend ten minutes with you to know what's wrong with you." He seemed so confident that I was taken aback. "Have you been taking antibiotics?" he asked.

"Yes," I replied. "I took them for several months because I had an eye infection."

"Bad, bad doctors!" he exclaimed. And he went on to ask, "And have you been taking hormone replacement tablets?" I nodded. For a year or two I had attended a menopausal clinic in a hospital in South London, hoping that it would help my condition.

"There you are," he said jubilantly, flinging his hands in the air.

"Well, what's wrong with me?" I asked impatiently.

"You've got Candida," he replied. I had never heard of it. "Wait a minute." He telephoned down to his receptionist. "Get in touch with Holland and Barrett's immediately and ask them to reserve a copy of *Candida Albicans...could yeast be your problem?*. Tell them that a lady will pick it up in half an hour. And bring up some nystatin."

"I've already taken nystatin," I said with considerable disappointment. "My own doctor gave me some."

"It was not powerful enough. The powder is much more powerful," he said and he went on to explain what had gone wrong. "You have friendly bacteria in the bowel, but if you take antibiotics for any length of time they destroy this friendly bacteria and a yeast fungus infection takes control, affecting all parts of the body. Does your stomach feel bloated?"

"Yes," I replied.

"You're a classic case of Candida Albicans," he said. "Let me look inside your mouth." He did so and pointed out the tiny white flecks on the inside of both my cheeks, which I had never noticed before and neither had any of the doctors or specialists I had consulted. "I had one patient who was so depressed—really suicidal—and her stomach was so bloated...it was out there," he said, illustrating with his hands. He stood up. "Listen," he went on, "I go all over the country lecturing, visiting hospitals and talking to specialists about Candida."

"But I've been to hospitals and seen specialists but nobody has ever mentioned it. Why?" I asked.

"Because only doctors who are well up know about it," he replied.

It was unbelievable, but it certainly seemed to be the case after what I had experienced in the hands of the medical profession.

The receptionist brought in the nystatin powder in a black cylindrical container.

"Take a ¼ teaspoonful in water four times a day and don't forget to swill it around your mouth," he advised.

I was excited by the fact that someone apparently knew what was the cause of my ill-health but little did I know that I had a long road to travel before being cured of that particular illness.

"Read the book," he urged. "You're an intelligent woman."

He gave me a chart to record everything I ate during the following week to see if my diet was acceptable and a list of all the forbidden foods. They were all foods containing yeast and refined carbohydrates because the yeast feeds on sugar. That in itself was a formidable array of foods and it looked very daunting. He handed me some literature he had on the subject of Candida and I quickly glanced through them. They listed case histories of people who had been cured of the illness by the use of the drug nystatin.

"Impressive isn't it?" he said, and I had to agree with him.

After making an appointment for the following week and paying him his fee and for the precious nystatin powder, I rushed to Holland and Barrett's to purchase the book called *Candida Albicans* by Leon Chaitow. As soon as I arrived home I read the book from cover to cover and over and over trying to assimilate all the information it contained.

It was the first insight I had had on the illness called Candida and it was a revelation to me. I now had a tried and tested programme to follow which would rid me of the terrible illness.

His was the non-drug approach to Candida, which I decided to follow along with the use of nystatin. It seemed that Dr Orion Truss in America was the first to pioneer research into Candida in 1979 and wrote a book called 'The Missing Diagnosis' which was unavailable in Britain at the time. He advocated the use of the drug nystatin to kill off the yeast fungus infection along with an anti-Candida programme. There are now other books available: one is called *The Yeast Connection* by Dr Crook. Through these books and literature I have since read on the illness I have learned that thrush is a yeast which transforms itself into a fungus which can root itself in the lining of your throat, stomach and bowels with telltale white flecks on the inside of your mouth.

A prolonged use of antibiotics, especially the tetrocyclines, which is what I used, can kill off the natural good bacteria in the bowel and the yeast can rapidly multiply and fill this vacuum and it is hard for the protective bacteria to reestablish itself—hence Candida Albicans. I read also that the yeast can travel right through the body from the mouth to the anus. It had done so in my case. But according to Dr Truss a stool culture test will not indicate correctly if an individual has a chronic yeast infection because yeast is natural to the body. Stool tests alone, it seems, have led to missed diagnoses. That is exactly what happened in my case, as you will see.

Leon Chaitow's book *Candida Albicans* in fact became my bible. I would refer to it endlessly. His anti-Candida programme consisted of eliminating all foods containing yeast, such as bread, biscuits and alcoholic beverages, plus the avoidance of refined carbohydrates because, as I have stated, yeast loves sugar. It is designed to starve the yeast fungus. I was also required to take Superdophilus, a potent friendly bacteria to re-establish residence in the bowel, because a deficiency of this can actually cause Candida, garlic capsules to cleanse the bowel, oleic acid (olive oil) which acts on the Candida plus a long list of vitamin and mineral supplements to build up my sadly depleted immune system. He also states that self-help is necessary until the medical profession becomes aware of the import of this knowledge. Until recently I belonged to a group called the 'Candida Albicans Group' especially formed to help sufferers, giving up-to-date information concerning the illness and a list of doctors who are prepared to help, but unfortunately it has to be private.

The medical profession can be so narrow-minded and stubborn in their attitude. They are indeed very slow and unwilling to accept new ideas. Candida is truly an illness of the twentieth century. I was obliged to suffer years of ill-health because doctors were ignorant of the illness, but even when I told them the nature of my illness, after it had been correctly diagnosed, I wasn't taken seriously, with the result that I was entirely on my own throughout, having to cope with a bewildering array of symptoms plus keeping strictly to a lengthy anti-Candida programme. It wasn't easy and I regard it as a miracle that I was eventually able to overcome that particular problem.

However, on with the story. Needless to say, I went again to the allergy clinic, but I don't know how I managed to get there. I felt so dizzy and disorientated and sick.

I spoke to the receptionist before I saw the osteopath and I told her how I felt. She seemed concerned and said, "If the osteopath can't help you, Dr McEwen can." I took note of what she said.

When I saw the osteopath and told him how sick I had been the whole week he advised, "Take the nystatin just before a meal and not on an empty stomach."

My sickness, of course, could have been caused by the Candida dying off, because it releases toxins which can have overwhelming symptoms in the body, but nobody mentioned that possibility.

I was given another chart and a list of further foods to avoid. The osteopath wanted me to eliminate wheat from my diet to see if I was allergic to it. It was yet another added burden but I was determined to comply with his wishes, even though to my knowledge I had never been allergic to anything in my life. However, Candida is known to cause allergies. Life, for me, was becoming a nightmare, what to eat and what not to eat was a real problem and when you felt as wretched as I did you haven't got the energy, spirit or will to sort it all out. I really don't know howl managed it. Perhaps it was meant to be so that I could record what happened.

Because the journey was so long and tiresome I didn't go again to see the osteopath. But, because I was feeling so ill, depressed and in desperate need of reassurance, a few weeks later I did telephone him.

"Do you remember me?" I asked timidly.

"Yes I remember you," he replied coldly.

"There's no improvement in my condition," I told him, "How long do you think I'll have to take the nystatin?"

"Some people have to take it for years," he said. "Look," he went on, "if my patients knew that I gave advice over the telephone while they have to pay for it they would be very annoyed." And with that he replaced the receiver.

He was not making any more money out of me and he clearly didn't want to know. I had telephoned him because he was the only person who I felt I could turn to for encouragement in battling with my illness and I felt that he had let me down very badly. If he had requested I would have gladly sent him a cheque in the post. Nevertheless, I am eternally grateful to him for correctly diagnosing my illness and guiding me on the long, long path back to health.

CHAPTER 7

I had my second colonoscopy at St. Thomas' hospital in January 1986, when another polyp was removed.

"We will keep a check on you," the young specialist said afterwards. "We'll see you in two year's time."

It was in fact three years later when I had another colonoscopy, when fortunately, nothing was found.

When I saw my usual specialist after the second colonoscopy to discuss the results with him, I took the opportunity of telling him that I had been diagnosed as having Candida, a yeast fungus infection, but he simply laughed and said, "Who told you that? If you had a fungus infection you would wither up and die." He was obviously not one of the well-up doctors the osteopath had referred to.

I was suffering from a severe bout of vomiting at the time and he prescribed gaviscon saying, "That will clear it up—it always does." Needless to say it did not.

I desperately wanted the telephone number of Dr McEwen, so I telephoned the allergy clinic and asked the receptionist if she would kindly give me the number. She was very reluctant to give it saying, "If I give you Dr McEwen's number the osteopath will not be able to treat you any further." I was not worried about that, so I persisted and she eventually gave in.

I rang the number as soon as I could but I was very disappointed to be told by his secretary that I would be unable to see him for a couple of months—not until June. So, I made an appointment for one afternoon in the middle of June.

At the first opportunity I told my GP that I had been diagnosed as having Candida and I told him about Leon Chaitow's book. He seemed interested and wanted to buy it. I pointed out to him the white flecks that were on my cheek inside my mouth and he exclaimed, "That's thrush!"

Before Christmas, because of my persistent vomiting, I had seen his colleague and he had given me ativan tablets. Since I had read about the dangers of those particular tablets I didn't take them.

The doctor noticed this on my notes. "If you take ativan tablets you'll have problems for the rest of your life," he said, shaking his head. But when I continued to have bowel and stomach problems, along with my so-called 'panic attacks', he too became fed up with seeing me.

"Nothing can be done for her varied symptoms until she has cured her anxiety," he told my husband who, in desperation, had telephoned him. But he was totally and utterly wrong. It was the Candida problem I had to overcome, which was a purely physical one.

On February 26th my relaxation and management classes began. They were to be held in a clinic a short bus ride from my home. But the moment I saw the other patients I knew I was completely out of place. There were six women and one man. Two of the women were only in their early twenties. It was obvious that they were suffering from some sort of psychosis or nervous illness.

In attendance were three psychiatric nurses—the nurse who had interviewed me, another young nurse and a man from Mauritius.

The aim was group therapy, and we all had to sit in a circle and tell the rest of the group all our problems, discussing it between us afterwards. One woman said that she had been taking ativan tablets for ten years. "I was on fifteen tablets a day for a few years but now they have managed to get me down to three a day."

I couldn't believe how anybody in their right mind would prescribe fifteen ativan tablets a day to a person for such a prolonged length of time. Whatever the reason it seemed an excessive dosage and the poor woman was now left with a terrible problem.

"If I knew they weren't a cure I would never have taken them," she sobbed. "I have panic attacks nearly every day. I even had one whilst crossing the road at the zebra crossing on my way to the clinic. It makes you feel you don't want to live anymore."

The nurses did their best to calm and encourage her, and because she couldn't cope with going out alone one of the nurses agreed to meet her and take her shopping the following day. I felt very sorry for her.

All the other patients had similar nervous problems; they couldn't cope with everyday life, whether at home with children or at work. The man couldn't hold down a job. Two of the women had agoraphobia and all of them seemed to suffer from panic attacks.

The nurses, of course, had merely been told that I was suffering from anxiety, but, knowing that my problems were physical and not the same as the rest of the group, I couldn't relate to any of them. There was no point in trying to explain my predicament to the group or even to the nurses; they would have just dismissed it as nonsense. So I just went along with everything and continued to attend each session for the number of weeks that it lasted. I did so just to please the OP who thought everything depended on the classes. But I could have told him that they would do no good whatsoever. I only wished it was that straight forward.

Nevertheless, during all that time I continued taking nystatin and did my best to keep to the anti-Candida regime as advocated in Leon Chaitow's book.

I still had a couple of months to wait before I could see Dr McEwen, so I decided to visit a South London clinic of natural medicine which I saw advertised in a health magazine. They mentioned that they did allergy testing and I was hoping they would be able to detect any allergies I might have, although I honestly thought that I didn't have any at that time.

I didn't know then that my panic attacks were in fact a classical symptom of allergic reaction and not, as the psychiatrists and GPs persistently kept telling me, the result of anxiety and nerves.

When I telephoned the clinic I spoke to a lady who stated, "The practitioner can diagnose what is wrong with you and then prescribe either a herbal or homeopathic medicine. It is called Bio-Energetic medicine. The first session lasts from one to one-and-a-half hours and it costs £5 6."

I made an appointment for the following week, even though at £56 for the first session I thought it rather expensive.

When the day came I arrived at the clinic on time for my appointment to be told that the practitioner was running late.

Meanwhile, the receptionist gave me some literature to read on the subject of Bio-Energetic medicine and I read them with interest. It seemed that the system of allergy testing at the clinic was within the field of Bio-Energetic medicine. A measurement taken at a special point on the hand with a stylus pen would show whether there is an allergy or sensitivity present. If the test proves positive then each item to be tested is placed in the test circuit and the allergy point is remeasured. If the first measure changes, the patient reacts to that substance. If it doesn't alter, then the substance doesn't cause reaction. In this manner 250 items can be tested.

The aim of the treatment was to raise the patient's tolerance to the allergens and strengthen or correct the organ function or weakness. This is done by the use of homeopathic preparations of the allergens themselves, so creating the opposite effect. I went on to read that Bio-Energetic medicine is based on the premise that illness cannot manifest itself from nowhere. Acupuncture, I read, is based on the concept of internal energy pathways connected to a special organ which can be influenced by the insertion of a needle at special points on each line.

These points, it seems, have low resistance and can be located electronically. Measurements can therefore be taken giving the energetic state of each specific organ so that it can diagnose an energetic function disturbance before it is followed by a chemical change and finally a pathological or diseased tissue change—the process taking years. But since these functional disorders can be discovered in the very early stages they can be treated before they progress too far. Again this was done by the use of a stylus pen on points on the hand and toes which gave a reading on a dial. Homeopathic, herbal or biological remedies are then tested by placing them into the measuring circuit to see if they have an impact on the patient and by changing the dosage or combination of remedies arrive at a unique and accurate prescription when the reading shows a normal balance. It all seemed very impressive.

Eventually, the practitioner, looking very smart in his blue jacket, came into the reception area. He apologised for keeping me waiting and then led me into a large room which had a black leather chair resembling a dentist's chair. The necessary electronic equipment was placed beside it. One wall had shelves that were filled with bottles of what I presumed were homeopathic or herbal medicine and another wall had a large diagram on it.

There was a lady assistant present. As soon as I entered the room I was asked to go into a small adjoining room where another lady in a white gown took a blood sample for testing.

After this I went back into the large room and the practitioner said, "Take off your shoes and stockings and sit on the chair."

When I had done as requested he lifted up the chair until my leg was outstretched and resting on a support. "what's the problem?" he asked.

I told him of all my health problems, about my visit to the osteopath and the fact that he had diagnosed that I was suffering from a yeast fungus infection called Candida. He was familiar with the illness.

"I take nystatin every day and follow the anti-Candida programme religiously," I told him.

"But did he test you for allergies?" he asked, and when I shook my head he heaved a sigh.

Then, for the next hour, he set about testing me. He pressed his stylus pen on various points on my hands and toes and every time it made a shrill noise. On each occasion he looked at the number on the dial, told his lady assistant who duly wrote it down. In that manner I was told I was being tested for all allergies and body malfunctions. He also tested each filling for possible mercury poisoning. Two of my teeth proved to have high levels of mercury release, which, incidentally, were removed later on, and a new filling called composite was put in its place.

At the end, when the testing was over, I was given a few small bottles by the practitioner who said, "I have given you the correct numbered homeopathic medicine. They will last you three weeks. Take the required drops of each medicine each day but don't drink coffee because it prevents the homeopathic medicine from working."

I was greatly disappointed not to be told of any possible allergies since that was the reason for my going there. Taking the correct numbered homeopathic medicine meant nothing to me and I was sure it wouldn't help greatly—if at all.

Before I left I was handed two small containers by the assistant who said, "One is for a urine test and the other is for a saliva test. Spit into it until you have filled it and bring it with you when you come next."

For an ideal state of health, blood, saliva and urine have certain numbers and any variation of these numbers represents a tendency towards disease and ill-health. Everything it seemed was based on numbers.

On the day of my next appointment I did my best to fill the small container with spit, but it proved to be a long and tedious task. You would be surprised how many times you have to spit to fill even the smallest container.

On that occasion, measurements of my blood, urine and saliva were taken and assembled. The practitioner then showed me on the chart that I was well off balance, which came as no surprise to me.

Once again he gave me homeopathic remedies. "I have to give you the correct number each time," he said.

I went a few times after that and he tested me on every occasion to see how I was progressing, giving me my homeopathic remedies, which I took unfailingly, but I didn't feel significantly better. In fact I was becoming more and more depressed, frighteningly so, with the result that I felt compelled to make an appointment at St Thomas' Hospital psychiatric clinic. When I telephoned them I stressed that it was an emergency and I was asked to go to Scutari. My husband drove me to the hospital and I waited there in a deplorable state. I felt sick, disorientated and in a much weakened state. I had lost two stone in weight.

A lady came up to me looking so bored by everything. She turned out to be the psychiatrist. I hadn't come across her before.

She led me into the same small room where I had seen the other very disagreeable psychiatrist and after going through the usual long list of questions as if it was really too much of an effort for her she said simply, "Well if you don't like amitriptylene you can have anafronil."

I just nodded. I felt too ill to question anything. "But they will make your legs shake," she warned.

"Oh God," I said to myself; "why does there have to be the inevitable side effects?" Nevertheless, I was determined to give them a try.

She wrote out a prescription and handed it to me, and as I got up from my seat she heaved a tremendous sigh. I really don't know what she was doing there. It seemed to me she was in the wrong profession and, alas, not long afterwards I was to encounter her again.

I took the prescribed anafronil tablets that night and the next morning my right leg shook so violently I didn't take them again.

In March, because of the Candida illness and the devastating effect it was having on my whole body, my immune system was so depleted that I caught the most terrible virus. I thought at the time I would never get rid of it.

The first signs I had of it was a blocked feeling in my ears. I had always suffered from an accumulation of wax in my ears but they had never felt like that before. It seemed as if they were full of gravel. I began using wax softener drops hoping it would soon clear up—it didn't. I made an appointment to see one of the panel of doctors and I saw an elderly lady doctor. She had come to the house on one occasion after I had had one of my so-called 'panic attacks'. She gave me valium to calm me down. I thought then that she was an extremely sensible and compassionate person but I was in for yet another shock.

I told her about the feeling I was having in my ears and she looked into them.

"Use a wax softener for a few days and then come to the clinic and the nurse will syringe them for you," she said abruptly.

"I've already used a wax softener," I told her.

"Well the nurse will do it for you straight away," she said and she quickly wrote on a slip of paper and handed it to me. Her whole attitude towards me had changed.

The nurse proceeded to syringe my ears and remarked afterwards, "Your ears look very red and inflamed on the inside."

I was surprised by her remark but I didn't take much notice of it until a few days later when I felt a vibration in my right ear, and I could also hear a high-pitched ringing sound. I began to get extremely worried about it, especially when some nights I woke up to find both ears ringing loudly—so loudly in fact that they had actually woken me up. I was also feeling very dizzy.

My appointment at the menopausal clinic was every six months and one was due in a few days' time. Though I had stopped taking the hormone replacement tablets because the osteopath had said they contributed to the Candida, I wanted to see if the doctor would be helpful with my newly acquired problem—the ringing in my ears and the dizziness.

The young doctor was very patient and concerned when I poured out all my problems. I told him how I was trying desperately to overcome the yeast fungus infection, Candida, which I was convinced had caused the new and very alarming problem—the ringing in my ears.

"I don't know where to turn to for help," I told him.

"I can't do anything for you here but I'm going to write a letter to King's College Hospital for you to see an Bar, Nose and Throat specialist. They can treat tinnitus today," he replied.

Tinnitus! I had never heard of the word before but, sadly, I was to be well acquainted with it later on. However, a week or two later when the appointment came for me to attend the Ear, Nose and Throat clinic at the hospital it wasn't until the middle of June, which was three months later. To me the length of time was ridiculous.

A few days after my visit to the menopausal clinic I developed a sore and inflamed throat and severe aching and a burning sensation all over my body, especially my back, which was aching so much I didn't know where to put myself. I tied a hot water bottle to my back hoping to get some relief but I was shaking from head to foot.

I felt obliged to call the clinic and I spoke to my usual OP, telling him about the sore throat and terrible aching, especially in my back.

"If you come to the clinic at 4 p.m. I can see you then," he said, having no intention whatsoever of visiting me. The thought probably never entered his head and I wondered how ill you would have to be before he would even consider it. I dreaded to think.

I drove myself to the clinic in the most terrible state and dragged myself up the flight of stairs to the waiting room.

The doctor got up from his chair when I entered his room and immediately snapped at me, "Bend forwards, bend sideways to the right, bend sideways to the left," all of which I tried to do. He went on to order, "Now get on the bed and lie on your stomach."

I collapsed on to the bed panting for breath. He came over to me and touched down my spine. 'There's nothing wrong with your back," he snapped. "Now get up and let me look at your throat."

I dragged myself up from the bed and managed to stand up. I opened my mouth for him to take a look and he said immediately, "You've got a virus. There's nothing we can do about a virus. Go home and go to bed."

That was the last time I went to him.

A couple of weeks passed and I didn't seem to be shaking off the virus at all. I had been gargling with salt water and the sore throat had eased, but I was still aching all over. I was dizzy and I still had the wretched ringing in my ears.

I had an appointment at the Gastrointestinal clinic at that time and I was determined to keep it—don't ask me why.

My husband drove me there in the car and parked in the car park on the Embankment. I walked on ahead of him but the walk from the car park to the hospital's Gastrointestinal clinic, through all the corridors, proved too much for me and the moment I arrived I collapsed on a chair with my head and arms resting on a table.

A nurse came running up to me.

"What's the matter? What's the matter?" she kept repeating. But when I didn't respond she went quickly into one of the doctor's consulting rooms and a young doctor came out of the room and walked over to me. He lifted my head up by my hair.

"What's the matter?" he asked.

I felt too ill to answer, so he said to one of the nurses,

"Bring her into my room."

Two of the nurses managed to get me up from the chair and walk me into the doctor's consulting room, where I was put on a bed and I lay there with my eyes closed.

The nurses began attending to me whilst the doctor was finishing with a patient in the adjoining room.

"Are you a diabetic?" one of the nurses asked.

"No," I replied emphatically.

"Then why did you collapse?" the other nurse asked.

"Oh, she always does that," the first cut in.

"I don't always collapse," I protested.

"Well, we'll check your blood just in case," said one of the nurses.

"I've got some sort of virus," I told them. "I should never have attempted to come here."

By that time my husband had arrived at the clinic and he was ushered into the room looking full of concern. I felt sorry for him. The doctor then came into the room and began to examine me. I told him that I felt extremely dizzy and weak. When the examination was over he ordered, "Get up and walk along that white line."

I struggled, with the help of my husband, to get up from the bed and very shakily I walked along the white line.

"There's nothing wrong with your balance," he said irritably. "I can't find anything wrong with you!"

He led us into the adjoining room and we all sat down.

"You can have a blood test before you go to test for B12 deficiency," he said.

He handed me the necessary slip and we both walked slowly to the haemotology department. I had been there several times in the past and the lady who took the blood sample recognised me.

"I've never seen you looking so ill," she said sympathetically. "If you can't get any satisfaction here why don't you go privately?"

I just nodded.

A few days later, my husband, at my request, drove me to the casualty department at St Thomas' Hospital. It happened to be on the same day as my appointment at the psychiatric clinic which I didn't intend keeping, regarding it as a waste of my time.

At the onset of the ringing in my ears I had gone there and the doctor on duty, after giving me a thorough examination, had said, "It's a virus. I knew that when you said you had ringing in the ears."

But, not surprisingly, on that occasion they refused to see me.

"No, we can't see you. You must see a specialist," the sister kept repeating, but when they realised that I had an appointment at the psychiatric clinic that very afternoon and desperately wanting to get me off their hands, they insisted that I kept the appointment. "The psychiatrist will arrange for you to see a specialist," the sister said. A specialist of what they didn't say!

Immediately they put me into a wheelchair and I found myself being wheeled through numerous corridors to the psychiatric department.

My husband followed. It had become a farcical scenario and if I hadn't been so ill I would have seen the funny side of it, but then I wouldn't have been there in the first place if I hadn't been so ill. And to cap it all I was obliged to see the lady psychiatrist I had seen several weeks before in Scutari.

She arrived at the clinic five minutes after I had arrived there and the nurse who had wheeled me there whispered something to her. Still in my wheelchair, I was taken immediately into her consulting room. My husband came with me. I felt so ill I nearly collapsed.

"How did you get on with the drug I gave you?" she asked in her usual bored manner. She always looked half asleep.

"My legs shook so violently in the morning after taking the pill that I didn't take any more," I replied.

She looked at me as if I was mad and, turning to my husband, she said, "I can see you've got a lot of problems with her."

I could have killed her. She had no idea how to treat a patient. She just rubbed them up the wrong way.

"Well, what about the prottraden?" she said with a sigh, turning to me.

"Every time I took them I woke up with a pain in my left arm,,, I replied which was true.

"They won't give you a pain in the arm," she replied, sneeringly. She was treating me as if I was a hopeless idiot. I wished someone had told her there was nothing wrong with my mind. But when she began talking exclusively to my husband, ignoring me completely, I became angrier and angrier until I finally erupted. "You just waste my time!"

"And you waste my time!" she shouted back. "I'm going to write to your GP."

"Yes, you do that," I snapped as I made for the door, still in my wheelchair. It was then that my husband wiped the floor with her and she stood there dumbfounded. She actually thought he would side with her. I'm afraid as a psychiatrist she was just one big joke!

My husband wheeled me back to the casualty department and I told the sister what had happened. She just shrugged her shoulders and said, "We can't see you here. You must see a specialist."

A week or two after my collapse at the hospital I telephoned the doctor's secretary to see if they had the results of my blood test—they hadn't. But when I telephoned the second time the doctor was in the room and his secretary said, "The doctor would like to have a word with you."

"You can't keep phoning my secretary," he snapped in his usual irritable manner. "She's very busy…you will be told the results when I see you at your next appointment."

"I hope I won't be seeing you," I retorted quickly. I couldn't help it.

A few weeks passed without the symptoms of the virus abating so I telephoned the doctor's clinic and asked to see the lady doctor. After the way the other doctor had behaved over the back episode I was determined not to see him again.

"You haven't got an appointment but I'll put you in. I'm sure she will see you," the receptionist answered.

I was obliged to wait in the clinic for a considerable length of time, as usual in the most lamentable state. Tears ran down my cheeks.

When my name was called I entered her room to be met by a scowling face.

"What can I do for you?" she said icily.

Immediately I burst into tears as I tried to explain how ill I felt, but she just grimaced and then, glaring at me, she said nastily, "We can't go on treating you," and she kept repeating it. That was her answer to my call for help. I couldn't believe anyone could be so callous. But when she could see that I was taking not the slightest notice of what she kept repeating she snapped, "Well what's the problem?"

I had already told her but I repeated my concern over the virus that just wouldn't go away.

"How do you know it's a virus?" she asked.

"I don't know it's a virus," I replied, "but that's what the other doctor said it was."

"Well viruses go when they want to go," she said. "But I'm not going to do anything now…not without an appointment." I didn't answer, I just sat there too ill to move. Tears again began to run down my face and she repeated her remark, "I'm definitely not going to do anything for you now…not without an appointment."

I honestly thought the woman must have been mad to make such a fuss over an appointment when I was already sitting in her consulting room. Later, however, I heard that she upset a lot of patients because of her unreasonable behaviour.

"I'm not going to do anything for you today," she repeated, "but if you make an appointment for Monday morning I will arrange for you to have a blood and urine test at the hospital."

I made an appointment for Monday morning, knowing that it would again prove to be a waste of time. I had had numerous such tests. However, when Monday came I went to the clinic and she gave me the necessary slips of paper to take to the hospital. "Make an appointment for Friday and I will let you know the results then," she said.

I went immediately to the hospital. My husband, as usual, was required to escort me there; otherwise I would never have been able to manage it. And, once again, I had a blood and urine test.

A few days later I telephoned the clinic and asked for the results. "They are both normal," I was told. It was what I had expected.

Nevertheless, I kept the appointment I had made with the lady doctor on Friday and I told her about the vibration and ringing in my ears. I still felt very ill but there was nothing, it seemed, she could do about that.

"You must see an Ear, Nose and Throat specialist," she said.

"I already have an appointment to see an Ear, Nose and Throat Specialist at King's College Hospital but it isn't until June," I told her.

"Then why don't you go privately? It only costs £30. I'll write a letter for you. You telephone the hospital and make an appointment and pickup the letter this afternoon," she said.

I did just that and was given an appointment to see an Ear, Nose and Throat specialist the very next day.

I arrived early for the appointment feeling so ill I could barely lift up my head.

The specialist, a rather seedy looking man, asked a number of questions and I told him all about my Candida illness and my desperate effort to get rid of it.

He looked into my mouth and said wearily, "There's no sign of fungus."

"Well what are these white specks on the inside of my cheek?" I replied, pointing them out to him.

"That's not fungus," he said, glaring at me. "I've seen many throats with fungus and that's not it."

I saw no point in mentioning it further.

"What's wrong with your ears?" he eventually asked.

"I have a vibration and a high pitched ringing sound in my right ear and my left ear rings occasionally," I told him.

"Well let's test your hearing," he said rather half-heartedly and I wished he would show more interest.

He put a plug in my right ear and he gave me something to hold which I was to press whenever I heard a sound. He then followed the same procedure with the left ear, but I had no difficulty in picking up sounds, however faint.

"Your hearing is perfect," he said afterwards. "Now let me look into your ears." He did so with a light and then with a shrug of his shoulders he said, "I can't find anything wrong with your ears, are they ringing now?"

I shook my head.

"Well then," he said, raising his eyebrows as if to tell me I was making a fuss about something that wasn't there.

He really was very frustrating, but I went onto ask, "Is it the Candida that is causing the ringing?" I was hoping for a little enlightenment.

"Oh there are many things that can cause it," he replied, nonchalantly. "What does your doctor say about ft?"

"Oh, all she says is that she can't go on treating me any more," I blurted out, really out of frustration with him.

But with that he rose from his seat and said, "Well I'm not going to be brought into any disagreement between you and your doctor," and he walked out of the room. Nothing the medical profession did surprised me any more.

My appointment with Dr McEwen was approaching. It was something I eagerly awaited. So was my appointment at King's College Hospital, but I wasn't expecting anything to come of that visit and I was proved correct.

Before that I had an experience with a hypnotist that is worth mentioning. It was early June and although I had recovered from the virus and the intense aching in the muscles had gone, I still felt very shaky and anything but well. My intestinal symptoms were not so severe, probably because of the nystatin I was taking and the anti-Candida regime I was trying to follow, but I still had a vibration and ringing in my ears and my so-called 'panic attacks'.

I made an appointment to see him and found that his Hypnotherapy Centre was in a room at the back of a shop.

He seemed pleasant enough when I told him of all my problems.

"We will go right back to your childhood, in fact before you were born," he said. And he went on, "Your present illness could be attributed to your thoughts and emotions over the years. It will take twelve sessions and you have to make a contract with me to keep those twelve sessions. In that time we will go right back and find the problem…what is causing your illness. One patient I had stammered very badly and we went back many years until I found out that he had at one time wanted to kill his father. When he realised his guilt was causing the problem he never stammered again."

I made an appointment for the following Tuesday.

"It's £25 in advance," he said, so without hesitating, I wrote out a cheque for £25.

The following Tuesday my husband drove me to the Hypnotherapy Centre and waited outside in the car whilst I went inside.

The hypnotherapist took me into his room and without saying a word he sat down at his desk and wrote out an appointment card and pushed it towards me.

"That's £25," he said.

That meant I was paying £50 without receiving any treatment and I didn't intend doing that, and furthermore it coincided with my appointment with Dr McEwen and I didn't intend missing that for anybody, so I simply said, "I'm afraid I can't come next week."

He just stared at me as if I was mad. He was completely dumbfounded and he bellowed, "Why can't you come next week? You've made a contract with me to come twelve times and you cannot break it."

"I have an appointment with Dr McEwen to find out about possible allergies," I replied.

"You would rather put Dr McEwen before me?" he bawled.

"I have waited months to see Dr McEwen and I don't intend missing it…furthermore, I don't intend paying for another session before I have even had the firs. I'd rather pay at the end of the session," I told him.

Immediately he began banging his fists on his desk. His face was flushed and he was totally out of control. "I'm not having you messing me up," he yelled as he continued to bang his fists on the desk.

I looked at him in horror and I could feel myself beginning to shake uncontrollably, but I managed to get up from my seat and walk out of the room. He followed me yelling, "You can't leave. You've made an appointment with me for twelve sessions."

I walked shakily to the car, parked close by, and told my husband what had happened. He went immediately to see the hypnotist who apologised profusely for his behaviour. "Bring her back and we'll try again," he said.

Needless to say, I didn't go back. He was more in need of treatment than I was.

As for my appointment at King's College Hospital, it turned out to be as expected. I was given the same ear tests as before, after which the consultant said, "Your hearing is perfect, so the ringing in your ears might go of its own accord. If they do get worse come back and see us."

My long awaited appointment with Dr McEwen finally arrived. My husband drove me to his clinic in Harley Street and I sat reading the magazines in the large waiting room whilst waiting to be seen. It wasn't long, however, before a genial, balding, middle-aged man appeared at the door.

"Mrs Barrett?" he called out.

"That's me," I said eagerly as I got up from my seat.

He beamed at me and led me into his small consulting room. He sat down at his desk and I sat opposite him. He beamed at me again and I said quickly, "My troubles are not because of allergies. I have never had allergies in my life."

"We'll see," he said pleasantly, and then he began asking me a multitude of questions concerning my condition, which I did my best to answer correctly.

I told him that I had been given his name and telephone number from another allergy clinic I had attended. He knew the osteopath concerned. I also told him what he had diagnosed

- Candida—and the fact that I was taking nystatin powder four times a day plus keeping to a yeast free diet.

"Nystatin takes the minerals out of the system," he said with concern, which was news to me, but he was probably correct.

"I also still have so-called 'panic attacks,'" I went on to tell him.

"You really must breathe properly," he said.

"I do breathe properly," I retorted. "I'm a trained singer."

I knew very well that that was not the reason for the panic attacks.

"You breathe shallowly," he said, shaking his head. "You must make an appointment to see this lady. She will show you how to breathe properly…but she does live quite a distance away."

He gave me the name and telephone number of the lady and I put it into my handbag, but I had no intention of contacting her.

"Now take off your jacket," he said. So I took off my jacket. "Now breathe deeply twenty times."

I breathed deeply twenty times and almost collapsed. My head was swimming.

"There, I told you…you're hyperventilating. You can give yourself angina that way," he said.

But I saw no point in the exercise whatsoever.

"I want you to go to Biolab and have a cytotoyic test for allergies. it involves a blood test and hair analyses. I also want you to have a sweat test. That will test for minerals in the body," he said.

It was all new to me. I had never heard of a cytotoyic test for allergies. At last something positive was being done I thought to myself.

"And don't forget to take a sample of tap water with you. I'm also going to ask for a special Candida test. That will cost you extra," he went on. "All in all it will cost you £120.

It seemed a lot of money but I would have paid anything.

He ticked the tests he wanted me to have on a green form and handed it to me saying, "Give this to Biolab. Telephone them right away and they will give you an appointment within three days. The results will come to me and also to you."

The test it seemed could only be taken through a doctor.

Before leaving, I was taken downstairs to the basement and a sample of blood was taken. I don't know what that was for—presumably it was another test for allergies. It cost £20.

"She's not being desensitized today," he told the gentleman who took the blood sample.

"I like to see people three weeks after they have taken the test," he said as we walked back upstairs and he warned, "but next time be prepared to wait a couple of hours. You were lucky today. I'm always ruling late."

That turned out to be only too true. However, with a beaming face he bade me farewell and waved good-bye.

I wrote out a cheque for his very substantial fee and for the blood test and gave it to the receptionist before leaving.

Immediately I arrived home I contacted Biolab and just as Dr McEwen had said I was able to make an appointment for three day's time. The test had to be taken about twelve or one o'clock, as late as possible, so that the blood would be fresh when it arrived at the laboratories in York in the evening. I was given strict instructions not to eat for twelve hours before the test and drink only mineral water in the morning. I was also not allowed to clean my teeth in the morning. All this I adhered to and I went to Biolab at the appointed time.

It was a very busy place and I waited patiently for my name to be called. I remember feeling like a wet rag as I sat there. I marvelled at people who were full of energy, people who smiled and those who appeared to be enjoying life. I was a world away from them. I simply struggled on from day to day.

When my turn came a very pleasant lady took a blood sample and then snipped a piece of hair from underneath at the back of my head. She told me to take off my jacket and blouse so that she could stick a large piece of plaster on my back. It was the sweat test. "That will show if you have any mineral deficiencies," she said.

Since I had to wait for 45 minutes with the plaster on, I decided to go and have some food and a cup of coffee at a nearby restaurant. Having had the blood sample taken I was now at liberty to eat and drink. I arrived back in time to have the plaster removed.

Days later the results of the test arrived. They were from the York Medical and Nutritional Laboratories and I couldn't believe what I read.

I had severe reactions from wheat, corn, egg, coffee and chocolate and moderate reactions from rice, beef, chicken, turkey, shellfish, peppers, mustards, banana, grapes and spinach. I was also suffering severe reactions from additives, but which numbered ones they didn't stipulate.

Both chlorine in tap water and Candida had given a severe reaction.

I kept staring at the results, completely shaken. All those allergies when all my life I had never ever suffered from any allergy.

To my added dismay I was very deficient in zinc and moderately deficient in magnesium.

In his book, *Candida Albicans*, Leon Chaitow had stated that Candida caused allergies and zinc deficiency was a common factor. Here was the proof, I thought to myself.

I didn't know why I wasn't responding quickly to the drug nystatin and a yeast free diet, but now I had even more to contend with. I had to eliminate even more foods from my diet. The problems seemed insurmountable and I despaired of ever getting well again.

I made another appointment to see Dr McEwen, but unfortunately he was going to be away in three weeks so I had to wait four weeks.

On that occasion, just as he had warned me, I had to wait for two hours after my appointed time. I found it very trying and went to a cafe' halfway through the waiting time. I drank a cup of tea because I was allergic to coffee!

After what seemed an eternity Dr McEwen came into the waiting room and called my name. He was his usual genial self, but I must have showed my irritation at being kept waiting for so long because he said, "I did warn you. You were very lucky last time."

On that occasion there was a young lady assistant present who walked in and out of the room. "She's a very allergic person," he said, "if I didn't desensitize her she would be flat on her back." The young lady nodded her head and smiled at me. "I've kept many people going for over twenty-five years. That's why I need the money—to keep the lab going. A lot of people depend on me. Do you know I earned over £100,000 last year and I didn't pay tax because it all goes to keep the lab going. You have to wait so long because I pack in as many patients as I can to earn the money."

I believed him. The lab was for research and for making his own particular desensitizing fluid.

On his desk lay the booklet from the York Medical and Nutritional Laboratories. He opened it and said, "You are not an allergic person. An allergic person would have many more foods listed positive than you have."

He seemed to have lost a little interest in me because of that fact, but he spent a great deal of time with me going over the results and making a chart on how to mask the allergic foods, such as eating a lot one day and then leaving it off for a week and alternating it with other allergens.

I looked on with interest but it was all too much for me to cope with at the time. Anyway, my aim was to get rid of the allergies and not mask them. I knew it was the Candida that was causing the problem.

"I have allergies and when we go abroad my wife says try so and so and I do, with the result that I am sick," he said, trying to console me. And he then added, "But I have a wonderful life."

"I've avoided all the foods listed and I've bought a filter for the tap water, but I still feel ill," I said despairingly and I asked about the possibility of being desensitized.

"I will desensitize you, but it's very expensive and you will be dependent on me for the rest of your life," he said. "If I do desensitize you it will take up to five months before it works. But I am confident that I will have you eating normally within two years." However, he didn't elaborate on how he was going to achieve it.

"I have never had allergies before," I said. "What is the cause of it? Is it the Candida?"

He paused for a moment and then said, "A colleague of mine says that if you take half a teaspoonful of nystatin three times a day for three months you will lose all your allergies." He shrugged his shoulders but I knew that was probably the answer to my problems and I told him I was prepared to increase my dosage of nystatin.

"Be careful," he said, "because nystatin takes all the minerals out of the system, and at the moment you have only half the zinc in your body that others have. Also the extra dosage might give you nausea and diarrhoea."

"I'm definitely going to take as much as I can tolerate," I told him.

"Well," he said, "I'd better keep a check on you." He got up from his seat and took a few boxes from a shelf and put them on his desk.

"I want you to take 10mg of zinc a day and these magnesium tablets, but a tiny dose of Epsom Salts will do for magnesium. Don't take enough to make you go to the toilet," he said with a smile. He also gave me multivitamin and mineral tablets free from allergens. "Don't take the nystatin anywhere near your meal times or your zinc and magnesium tablets," he urged and I promised to heed his advice. He then gave me a box of nystatin powder saying, "I do it for £10," which was £5 less than the osteopath had charged.

He gave me a booklet called *Enzyme Potentiate Desensitization* and said, "Read it thoroughly and let me know if you want to be desensitized." He also gave me a leaflet called The Psychological Irritable Bowel Syndrome, but I had been through all that before. "Make an appointment for three month's time, but be prepared to wait another couple of hours," he said.

I had been worried about the possibility of going abroad and having to contend with all my allergies and he gave me a prescription for nalcom saying, "Take it as prescribed, it will stop the allergies." I never used it and still have the prescription.

As soon as I reached home I read carefully the booklet he had given me. It was his own particular method of desensitization. I read that a plastic cup was placed on your arm or thigh which first had been scarified to remove the waterproof layer of the skin. It was then held over the scarification for twelve hours. The desensitized fluid contains small doses of allergen extract together with a small quantity of beta glucoronidase especially prepared and activated. Beta glucoronidase is an enzyme present in all parts of the body and with this enzyme you could give smaller doses of allergens than in conventional Infections, hence the name. Frequency of the treatment depended on the nature of the allergens.

I decided immediately that it was not for me and dismissed it totally from my mind.

I then set about taking a higher dosage of nystatin and keeping strictly to my diet of avoiding yeast foods and refined carbohydrates, plus all my so-called allergens and taking a multitude of vitamin and mineral supplements. It was certainly a daunting task.

By that time I had removed my medical cards to yet another clinic closer to home. I hadn't been told to leave but I couldn't forget how callously they had behaved towards me when I felt so ill and desperately in need of help. Her words, "We can't go on treating you," had stuck in my mind. It was unforgivable.

The new clinic had three doctors, two female and one male. They were all very young. I made an appointment to see one of the ladies, a Miss Knight (not her real name). It was just after my appointment with Dr McEwen and they had received a letter from him. He had promised to write to them. But regarding the letter, which no doubt mentioned my allergies, she said, "We are conventional doctors and there are some doctors who don't believe in allergies and I must warn you that there are a lot of people who take advantage of the situation and are just out to make money. But Dr McEwen seems quite genuine."

"But I had a blood test, hair analyses and a sweat test at Biolab," I told her. "And the results came back from the York Medical and Nutritional Laboratories. They say they are 80% correct."

She looked distinctly unimpressed.

"Anyway," I went on, "I have been told that I am suffering from Candida and that is causing my allergies."

She refuted that idea at once with a sneer. "Have you had a stool test?" she asked.

"Yes," I answered, "but the experts say it doesn't show up in a stool test because it is natural to the body."

"It does show up," she retorted immediately, "I'll arrange for a stool test for you and we'll see."

"I'm taking nystatin for the Candida," I told her.

"But Dr McEwen says it takes all the minerals out of the body," she replied.

"He did say to take it well away from meals and my zinc and magnesium tablets—but I still have to take it," I told her.

She couldn't understand that and when I asked if she could prescribe the powder for me she replied hastily, "I could only do that if I thought you needed it—which I don't. If I did I would be struck off the register and I don't intend doing that for you."

She was totally and utterly ignorant of the real situation. She didn't have a clue. And when I mentioned the ringing, which was now in my head as well as my ears, she said, "When I was in Medical School they said that ringing at the top of the head was psychological."

Her remark was predictable. Anything that couldn't be explained had to be psychosomatic.

My stool was sent to St Thomas' Hospital for examination and when I rang up to ask for the results a week later I was told that it was completely normal in every respect. But then that is what I had expected.

CHAPTER 8

One day in early July I was browsing through a health magazine when I saw an advert for a book called 'Eliminate your Allergies', which could be obtained from The Institute of Advanced Health Research. The small print stated that there was no more need for special diets, desensitizes, nutrients or drugs. It stated 'How to discover for yourself and others the cause of your allergies and to correct them'. Naturally I was curious and eager to contact The Institute of Advanced Health so that I could be given more information. A man answered.

"I saw your advert in a health magazine and I would like to know more about it," I said. "I am suffering from various food and chemical allergies."

"It might be caused by an infection called Candida," he replied, without any hesitation.

"Yes," I said eagerly, "I've been told that I have a Candida problem. Can you cure it?"

"Yes," he replied. "We use the cube. The cube will do it. We've been using it for three years. We send them all over the world. Just send us a photograph and a list of your symptoms; then we will test to see if you are positive."

"What does that mean?" I asked.

"It means that if you are positive the cube can help you," he replied.

"Have you had any successes?" I asked.

"Yes," he answered. "We had one woman who had total allergies."

"And was she cured?" I asked, my optimism mounting.

"She's now eating normally," he replied.

"How long did it take?" I went on to ask.

"Five months," he replied.

"Well I'm definitely going to buy one," I said.

"Then I had better send you our catalogue. I'll send it today," he replied.

"How much is the cube?" I enquired.

"We hire them out for £10 a month," he replied.

"But how much are they to buy?" I went on to enquire. But he evaded the question. Perhaps he thought the price would be inhibiting.

"I'll put a catalogue in the post for you today," he said. "Look for the last page, it will tell you all about the cube."

"Yes that's fine," I replied and we left it at that.

The catalogue duly arrived the following morning and, just as the man had said, the back page told me all about the cube. It was all very complicated and I didn't pretend to understand at all, but I was certainly intrigued.

I read that the cube was literally a glass cube, a revolutionary healing device capable of treating and preventing an unlimited number of clinical conditions. It went on to say that the cube was a 24-hour a day therapist dedicated to your needs and backed by the most sophisticated laboratory of therapies put together in what is called a Workstation held at The Institute of Advanced Health Research. It seemed that the cube contained all the Logo of this work and was charged up with all the signals in the Workstation. I went on to read that the cube could be tuned to one individual and it then would commence to transmit any number and combination of required signals to any location on the first seven levels of the body. The seven levels were defined as L1—the entire physical body, L2—all forms of energy, L3—all kinds of feeling and emotion, L4—thought/mind, L5—insight/self awareness, L6—relationship projection of self, L7—perception/awareness of others. It stated that each level is as complex as the physical body and is a literal measurable signal differentiated only by the waveforms frequencies involved. It stated that it was unique because it could rid the body of residual trauma, i.e. all the problems from illnesses you had had throughout your life. It went on to state that when an illness was coming out you suffered slightly from the same symptoms for a few hours or days. Ml that was needed was a photograph and the cube could be tuned to me personally. But first you had to be tested for effectiveness.

I was still desperate for help and decided to give it a try and immediately found a small photograph of myself. I then wrote a letter to the Institute listing all my symptoms, which included stomach and bowel problems, a tight feeling in the chest with palpitations, dizziness and balance problems, plus nausea and a list of allergies to food and chemicals, but I deliberately didn't mention the ringing in my head and ears, fearing that it would complicate matters.

I posted the letter plus photograph to the Institute of Advanced Health Research that day and prayed that I would be tested positive so that I could soon be in possession of a cube.

In my eagerness I telephoned the Institute late afternoon the following day. This time a lady answered. And with a pounding heart I asked, "Have you tested my photograph yet?"

"I'm afraid we haven't got around to testing it yet. We only received it this morning. Telephone in a day or two," she replied patiently.

The next time I telephoned them was on Wednesday July 23rd, which happened to be the wedding day of Prince Andrew to Miss Sarah Ferguson. I remember it well because I watched the wedding on television. I telephoned them in the morning about 9.30 a.m.

"Have you tested my photograph yet?" I asked anxiously.

"Yes," she replied. "It tested positive."

I gave a huge sigh of relief. "Tell me how long it will take," I said, "and I will either buy or rent a cube."

"Five months," she replied. "How much are they?" I asked.

"It costs £110 plus VAT to buy a glass one and £100 to buy a wooden one," she replied.

"What's the difference?" I asked.

"The glass one is prettier and faster," she replied.

"Does it really work?" I asked with incredulity.

"We wouldn't be in business if it didn't," she answered sweetly.

"I'll send a cheque right away," I told her.

I posted the cheque immediately and the following day I rang them again. This time a man answered, "We are sending the cube to you today," he said.

"When will it begin to work?" I asked.

"It's already working," he gleefully replied, and then he soberly warned, "you're in for some rough patches."

"Shall I eat the foods I am allergic to?" I asked. "Not yet—make it easy on yourself," he answered. The cube arrived the following day, neatly packed in a black cylindrical box along with further instructions for cube owners and a long diagram called 'The Symbol of Completion' on which I could test to determine my progress in eliminating residual trauma on all seven levels. This was to be done by using the Body Tuning technique which was a simple muscle test. I was to touch, with a finger of my free hand, a numbered segment on the diagram whilst the other arm is tested for any weakness. The assistance of another person is needed. One hand rests on the shoulder, the other on the wrist, and the person doing the testing presses down the horizontal arm.

If it significantly weakens then it means a yes or positive answer. There was also an OUT symbol which I was to hold faced into the palm touching the area where I was experiencing the symptom while the other arm was tested for any weakness. A weak arm was a 'Yes' answer. That way I would be able to tell whether it was a new problem or residual trauma coming out. But it was all too much for me to cope with at the time and when next I telephoned the Institute I said to the lady who answered, "I doubt whether I shall be able to do my own testing."

"We don't usually have people coming to us cold. They usually come by word of mouth and are familiar with Body Tuning. We've only been advertising for the last couple of months. Give us a ring in 2 to 3 weeks time and we will do the testing," she replied.

"How can I find out about Body Tuning?" I asked.

"It tells you all about it in the book, 'Eliminate your Allergies,'" she replied.

"Well would you please send me a copy?" I asked, and she agreed to do so immediately.

The book duly arrived and I read it with considerable interest. I now knew the names of the people I was dealing with—Stephen and Mmdi Kane and it was Stephen who had written the knowledgeable book, greatly assisted by Mmdi.

Two weeks passed and I decided to telephone the Institute. All my symptoms were still with me plus an added one, intense aching all through my body. Some days I was free of it but others I ached so much I could barely get up from a chair. Incredible as it may seem the cube was having a definite effect on my whole body.

"Would you please let me know how I'm progressing? I've been on the cube for two weeks now," I told Stephen.

"You want your scores," he answered. "We'll do that for you tonight. Give us a ring tomorrow."

"Do you know what's wrong with me?" I asked.

"We always know what's wrong with a person," he replied, a little impatiently. "Give us a ring tomorrow."

When I called him the next day he said, "Candida is causing your allergies and you've got fractured chakras on levels 5, 6 and 7. Do you know what that means?"

"Yes," I replied. Chakras, I knew, were forces that energized the body.

"You are clear on levels 5, 6 and 7 and you are on segment 5 on levels 1, 3 and 4," he said. And then added sympathetically, "You are on the worst part—eliminating residual trauma from the deepest levels." By that he meant the physical level.

I was indeed suffering, but I felt it would all be worthwhile if the cube could eliminate all infections from my body including the wretched Candida.

However, I had no intention of abandoning my daily ritual of taking nystatin, plus Superdophilus and keeping strictly to my anti-Candida programme.

After five weeks on the cube I again telephoned the Institute to enquire how I was progressing.

"Ring back about 6 p.m. and we will give you your scores," Mmdi replied. And when I did so Mmdi said, "You are on segment 5 on levels 1, 2 and 3, and you are clear on levels 4, 5, 6 and 7."

"What is level 2 and 3?" I asked her, remembering only that level 1 was the physical level.

"Level 2 is the energy level," she replied, "and when it is on segment 5 you'll feel tiredness. Level 3 is the emotional level."

"My heart is beating very rapidly," I told her, "and I'm severely aching all over."

"Rapid beating of the heart is a classic allergy symptom," she replied. "When Candida is coming out you'll experience allergies. Use your arm test to see what exactly is coming out."

"You know I can't do that," I said.

"We'll test to see what is coming out," she replied, "and I'll give you a ring if it's anything to worry about."

I didn't hear from them so I assumed everything was progressing as it should be.

My right leg began to ache so much that I was begriming to drag it along behind me. I looked as if I had a limp. But I still intended to persevere with the cube.

Nevertheless, after seeing an advert for an allergy clinic in Bayswater, I decided to have a talk with the man running it—a Dr Hibberd who, to my surprise, answered with a pronounced Australian accent.

0"I've kept off all the foods I am allergic to but I'm still feeling very ill," I told him.

"Oh dear," he said sympathetically. "I do my own testing."

"I'm not really an allergic person, but they say I've got Candida," I said.

"Well I'm on the board for Candida research in this country. I'm a qualified doctor and you'll get the most up-to-date treatment that is available," he replied.

I was thrilled to find a doctor who actually recognised and was familiar with the devastating illness and I was determined to see him.

"Could I please make an appointment to see you as soon as possible?" I asked.

"I am booked up for weeks ahead," he said, "but I have a cancellation at 2 p.m. on Thursday. Would you like to come then?"

"Yes, that's fine," I replied.

"You'll go away with desensitization drops...a very important part of the treatment," he said. Then added, "Don't eat anything for four hours before coming and drink only mineral water."

I deliberately refrained from mentioning the fact that I was on the cube in case he thought some nut case was telephoning him.

On the day my husband drove me to the flat which was in the basement of a three storey house in Notting Hill. The door was opened by a bespectacled man in his early forties.

"You're early," he said, "I'll be through in a few minutes."

I sat in the hallway until a middle-aged lady emerged from his room and left. Dr Hibberd then came out and escorted me into the tiny room and once we were both seated began questioning me thoroughly on all aspects of my illness, making notes of my answers. I told him I had been diagnosed as having Candida by the osteopath at his North London Allergy Clinic and I went on to tell him of my visit to Dr McEwen and the results of my recent allergy test and sweat test. "My allergies are caused by the Candida," I told him and he nodded in agreement.

It was a relief to find a doctor who listened to what I had to say and actually understood the situation.

He placed a book called *Kinesology* on his desk and asked, "Have you heard about this method of testing?"

"Yes," I replied. I knew it was a muscle testing technique similar to Body Tuning, but not so sophisticated.

He told me to stand up and hold my right arm at shoulder height. He then took a small container from a shelf laden with containers, all of which were labelled. He gave it to me and told me to hold it in my left hand. He then put one hand on my shoulder and held the wrist with the other. In this manner he tested my arm for resistance to pressure. It held firm.

"You're no longer reacting to wheat," he said. "How long have you been off it?"

"Nine weeks," I replied.

He nodded. "Yes, it takes about ten weeks after abstaining from a food for the allergy to go. If you are still reacting to it after leaving it off for up to three months you can forget about it," he said.

In the same manner he went on to test my arm for any weakness whilst I held a number of containers. He seemed very skilled at the muscle testing technique and I was impressed because I had never seen it in action before.

He tested me holding a container labelled coffee and my arm weakened. "You're still reacting to coffee," he said, shaking his head.

I held another container and when he put pressure on my arm it significantly weakened. I looked down quickly to see what I was holding. The container was labelled 'Candida'.

"You shouldn't look at the labels," he said quickly, trying to prevent me from panicking too much. But he added reluctantly. "You've got it badly."

"Is there a way out of this?" I asked, simply.

"Oh yes," he replied, with conviction, "give it three to four months. There's an epidemic of Candida. The lady who just left is a nurse and she's got Candida." He added, shaking his head, "It does terrible things to the nervous system."

"I know that only too well," I said. "They sent me to a psychiatrist."

He closed his eyes in dismay.

"But I've been taking nystatin for over five months and I'm still suffering," I sighed.

"The trouble was that you took the nystatin but you didn't build up your immune system sufficiently," he replied, which was probably true. I have since read that people think that they can eradicate the spread of Candida just by taking large doses of nystatin, completely forgetting that it is the immune system that has broken down and needs to be built up. It is the body's defence system.

"Have you been taking a potent acidophilus?" he asked.

"Yes," I replied, "I've been taking Superdophilus."

He seemed pleased. And we went on then to discuss my recent sweat test.

"I have half the zinc in my body that normal people have," I told him.

"That's always the case," he replied, shaking his head. "How much zinc are you taking?"

"10mg a day," I replied.

He put a number of zinc capsules into a container and tested my arm. When he had found the right dosage my arm significantly weakened.

"You haven't been taking anywhere near enough zinc. You need seven pills of 50 mg each for a time," he said.

I thought it a bit excessive but was prepared to go along with what he advised.

"What dosage of nystatin are you taking at present?" he asked, and I told him.

"You must also increase the dosage of nystatin," he said after testing for the right amount. "It will go quicker."

"I may not be able to tolerate it," I replied, "but I'll try."

He then went on to test me for the correct dosage of all the supplements which were needed to build up my immune system.

"Your pancreas is overworked," he said, putting pancreatic pills along with the multitude of vitamin and mineral supplements he had piled upon his desk. I was also advised to take garlic capsules, the animo acid, oil of Evening Primrose and the oelic acid, olive oil. He also advised me to douche with Orithrush for yeast vaginitus.

"You have to take this high dosage of all the supplements for a while and then we'll gradually reduce them," he said. Then added, "We do the same for AIDS patients."

I was also given Caprystatin, the fatty acid, which is not available in Britain. Dr Hibberd had had it sent over from America. I had read about its effectiveness in the book *Candida Albicans* by Leon Chaitow and I was very pleased to have a further aid in my battle against Candida.

He tested my blood for hypoglocaemia and advised, "Leave off sugar. I never have it."

I was given a leaflet on the yeast foods barred to me, and a leaflet on hypoglocaemia.

"Do you want another cytotoxic test?" he asked. "I can arrange for you to have one free of charge and because I'm on the research team I can arrange for you to have one tomorrow."

I welcomed the opportunity of having a further allergy test to see how I was progressing, but I said sadly, "I can't manage to get there on my own."

"I'll arrange for taxis to take you there and bring you back," he replied, and he immediately rang the laboratory in Putney and an appointment was arranged for 10 a.m. the following morning.

"Don't eat for twelve hours before the test and only drink mineral water in the morning," he said.

I had asked to be given six week's supply of all my supplements to make sure I had enough to last me until my next appointment. He wanted to see me in a month's time but my husband would be abroad at that time and I was unsure whether I could manage to get to the flat on my own.

He put all the containers into a plastic bag and totalled up the cost.

"It comes to £276 and that includes my fee," he said.

I was staggered at the cost and I must have showed it because he went on, "You need all of it to build up your immune system. It will be less next time when we begin dropping the dosage."

I wrote out a cheque thinking, "What if I couldn't afford to pay for it all? Would I be doomed to live the rest of my life with Candida?" It was certainly a frightening prospect and, judging from the 'help' I had received from my GP and the hospital I attended it was, indeed, very likely.

I had mentioned the vibration and ringing in my ear to Dr Hibberd but he just dismissed it saying, "It's the Candida." However, it was becoming more and more of a worry. I had recovered from the virus and was hoping that that too would soon go, but it had remained persistent.

When I reached home I did as Dr Hibberd had instructed and telephoned the laboratories in Putney. They gave me the instructions I had to follow.

Next morning the taxi arrived at the house on time and I was taken to the laboratories. A young black lady took a blood sample and said the results would be sent to Dr Hibberd. Alas, I had automatically cleaned my teeth that morning forgetting completely that I was not supposed to. The lady made a note of it because she said it would significantly alter the results of the test.

A few days later I telephoned the laboratory and enquired about my results and I was told, "You had numerous allergies but because you used toothpaste that morning we put a blank on it. You're down to just a few now."

I was grateful for that.

I waited another few days and then telephoned Dr Hibberd. He had received the results of the test and very kindly gave them to me over the telephone. To my surprise I was no longer reacting to wheat, corn, coffee, chocolate and egg, but yeast and milk had come up positive.

Therefore, it seemed I still had Candida problems and I religiously continued to take the required dosage of all the supplements given to me by Dr Hibberd along with my nystatin and Superdophilus. I didn't take as much nystatin as Dr Hibberd had advised. I was afraid I would-n't be able to tolerate it, having already enough problems to cope with.

Meanwhile, believe it or not, I was still struggling with the cube and my aching was pretty consistent. I was obliged to drag my right leg after me now at all times.

I telephoned the institute regularly to find out how I was progressing and when I telephoned them after I had been on the cube for nearly two months, Stephen said encouragingly, "You're free on levels 4, 5, 6 and 7, but you have Chakra fractures on levels 5 and 6 and it will be much slower because you have them."

"I'm still severely aching all over," I told him.

"When Candida is coming out it feels as if your whole body is inflamed," he replied. "Don't worry, you'll be ail right," he added, obvi-ously sensing my acute distress.

The cube was certainly having a devastating effect on my body and there were days when I felt I could cope no longer. I used to cry a lot and pray that one day I would be free of it all.

Six weeks after my first visit I saw Dr Hibberd again. I was sufficiently well enough to travel there by tube although, because of the cube, my legs ached tremendously. He went over the results of my allergy test and then tested me, using the same muscle test, for the correct dosage of the necessary supplements. He again took a blood sample and tested it for hypoglocaemia saying, "It's good you've kept off sugar."

The cost of all the supplements was only fractionally less than before but I wasn't concerned about that so long as it would aid my recovery.

I told him I would visit him again in a few month's time. He had wanted to see me regularly once monthly but I felt I couldn't cope with the journey all those times.

As it turned out I didn't see him again, because by that time, something terrible had happened to me. Nevertheless, through it all I followed the anti-Candida regime as best I could, sending away to the manufacturers myself for all the necessary supplements.

I still continued to persevere with the cube, telephoning the institute regularly to ask for my scores. After I had been on the cube for about three months I asked how my infections were progressing.

After testing for me Stephen said, "There is no Candida anywhere in the body, but there is a streptococcus infection coming out."

"Well if you found no Candida in the body does that mean that I can eat anything?" I asked.

"No," he replied decisively, "because a streptococcus infection causes allergies."

I couldn't win it seemed.

"Have we put an energizer on you?" he then asked.

"No," I replied.

"Would you like that?" he asked.

"Yes," I replied enthusiastically. "How will it help me?"

"It will give you more energy to cope," he replied. "It usually quickens things up. I'll do it right away."

A few days later I received a letter from them informing me that they had put an energizer on me free of charge for a fortnight. But during that time I had yet another sore throat and I telephoned the Institute to ask their advice. Mindi answered. "It sounds like something coming out," she said. "Have you used Teatre? It's a homeopathic remedy. It is very good and you should be able to get it from a good homeopathic shop. Let us know if it doesn't get better."

I promised to do that and then pleaded, "Don't turn off the energizer."

"Oh, we can leave it on for another week," she replied.

Not long afterwards I telephoned them again and this time I spoke to an assistant.

"Why am I aching so much?" I asked.

"It's Candida coming out," she replied.

"But last time I telephoned, Stephen said they couldn't find Candida in the body," I protested.

"Oh well that's it. You know you are being healed. I had allergies and was a patient at the Institute before they used the cube. I have been on the cube for several months now. One man whose legs ache so much they go blue," she answered.

It was no comfort to me, however, and in my diary the following day I wrote, 'Aching so much—unable to move.' For Saturday and Sunday I wrote, 'Washed out,' and on Monday I wrote, 'Head dizzy and falling over—aching limbs, stomach trembling and a fast beating heart.' It was all really too much for anyone to cope with.

I telephoned the Institute and Stephen answered.

Immediately I began to cry. "Stay with friends for a few days," he suggested. But, alas, that was not possible. And he ended by saying, "Telephone tomorrow and by then we will let you know what's going on."

It was Mmdi who answered the following day. "You've got a type 3 stress, the worst. It's an environmental stress. You'll be groggy for a few days," she said.

"Oh God," I murmured. "I can't take any more." Nevertheless, I ordered an energizer hoping it would help. I received it a few days later. It was made of glass and pyramid shaped.

However, soon afterwards I was forced to telephone them again and tell them of the intense aching all over my body.

"You know," Stephen replied, "some people on the cube only experience headaches and most people have patches when they feel very well. But I've been through it all myself. I used to be a very allergic person, having very bad reactions. I would instantly collapse on the floor. I went on the cube and ached all over—just like you I ached so much I couldn't walk…but it was worth it because now I can eat anything."

"You were on the cube?" I questioned in surprise.

"Of course," he replied. "We tried it on ourselves first."

"Will it take as long as five months?" I asked, praying that he would say it wouldn't.

"If that's what we said," he replied. "It usually takes that length of time. Telephone us tomorrow and we'll let you know what's happening."

I couldn't wait for tomorrow to come, and when it did I telephoned again.

Stephen answered. "We've put you on another device to ease the aching muscles. It's not Candida coming out as we thought; it's the healing of the Chakras 5 and 6. That's the worst of the lot. Have you heard of the Chakras? There are lots of books on it," he said.

"Yes, I know about Chakras," I told him. "But what about my Candida?"

"We can find no Candida in your body. People think that everything is Candida but there are a lot of other things. By the time you come to the healing of the Chakras all the infections have cleared up. It's the worst of the lot," he repeated.

"My whole head is ringing," I told him, mentioning for the first time the ringing in my head and ear along with the vibration.

"It's the nerves in the head—it's working from the head down," was his reply.

"I have to stick it out," I said simply.

-280"I would," he ended by saying. I didn't worry too much about the aching, I knew that would eventually go—it was for me a definite result of being on the cube, but the ringing in my ears concerned me greatly. I didn't want to have to contend with that possibility for the rest of my life, I simply could not cope with it.

A little later on I telephoned the Institute and asked about the ringing in my ears, which by that time I knew was called tinnitus. "The signals are not strong enough for that," Mmdi replied, somewhat curtly. "Perhaps in the future."

CHAPTER 9

Again I found myself all alone trying to cope with a very distressing condition. This time it was tinnitus. The severe virus I had caught in April must have damaged my ears in some way.

I knew it would be a waste of my time but I went to discuss the problem with a GP. On that occasion I saw the young male doctor. All he had to say on the subject was, "Why don't you join a Tinnitus Group." He seemed unsympathetic and totally disinterested.

As I was leaving the surgery, I picked up a leaflet on tinnitus which was lying on a table. In large print was 'What is Tinnitus?' and underneath in smaller print it stated, 'Noises in the ear and head that don't appear to have any cause.'

When I arrived home I read the leaflet thoroughly. It seemed a new group was forming in the vicinity and the name and address of the person to contact was given. For more information I was to contact the British Tinnitus Association.

I rang the British Tinnitus Association and told them I was a tinnitus sufferer, but what they had to say was anything but encouraging. "Is there no cure?" I asked in dismay.

There was no reply.

"Well, does it go on its own?" I persisted.

"Sometimes it does," the gentleman replied.

"I've heard that acupuncture can cure it," I said optimistically, having read it somewhere.

"We have no knowledge of any person with tinnitus being cured by acupuncture," he replied.

My heart sank. "My God," I murmured, "is there no hope?"

"There are various groups of tinnitus sufferers. We'll send you a list along with our Newsletter," he said.

I gave him my name and address and thanked him.

I then telephoned the number given on the leaflet and was told by the lady that a new tinnitus group was to be formed and the first meeting was to be held a few weeks hence. She promised to write to me giving me all the details.

A few days later, as promised, I received the Newsletter from the British Tinnitus Association, plus the names and telephone numbers of the leaders of the various tinnitus groups in London. But what I read in the Newsletter wasn't very encouraging. There appeared to be no known conventional cure for tinnitus. I couldn't believe it, but that was the case. It was very depressing and in my anxiety I began to telephone the leaders of the various groups, hoping against hope for some assurance that all would be well. I ended up being in an even more desperate state.

One of the group leaders was a lady with a cultured voice.

"I have a vibration and a high-pitched ringing in my right ear," I told her.

"How long have you had it?" she asked.

"I've had it for five months now," I replied.

She sighed heavily. "They say it takes about five months to come to terms with it, and if you've only got a little in one ear," she said sadly. Her condition was obviously much worse than me.

"Have you tried acupuncture?" I enquired. "I've read that sometimes it can cure tinnitus."

"The acupuncturist I went to told me that it was a waste of time," she replied, and then added, "only cases that respond to osteopathic manipulation can be cured. I've got a masker, it sounds like a train coming into a station."

My heart plummeted. It wasn't what I wanted to hear. I couldn't think of anything more terrible.

She then went on to tell me of some of the people who had come to her group, "I had one boy of twenty-four, he was totally devastated. And there was another gentleman whose ears rang so loudly he couldn't hear the television," she said. And sensing my distress she added, "I' 11 give you the name of my consultant. He's the best in the country. See him and he will be able to tell you what is causing it."

"What's the good of that if they can't cure it?" I retorted, my anxiety mounting. "I want a cure."

"Oh, they can't cure it, but it's nice to know what's causing it," she replied.

That was a hopeless situation as far as I was concerned. Nevertheless, she gave me the name and telephone number of the consultant, Dr Jonathan Hazel. His practice was in the West End, near Harley Street. I had read articles written by him in the Newsletter sent to me by the British Tinnitus Association. He was indeed an expert on the subject but, alas, he offered no cure. After our conversation, however, I made an appointment to see him, but I had to wait until the middle of December which was three months away.

Still not deterred, I telephoned the leader of another group. She, it seemed, was an elderly lady. "My husband had it badly for fifteen years," she said.

Immediately I began to cry. I couldn't bear to hear any more. "I can't cope," I sobbed.

"I don't want to be a cripple in bed and nearly blind," she said softly, "but that's how I am now."

I went on sobbing away and she did her best to comfort me, saying, "God bless you, my dear."

Afterwards I just sat down and cried my heart out.

Nevertheless, I was still determined not to give up all hope—not yet anyway—I would try everything, including acupuncture—it couldn't possibly do me any harm.

I had read that the only harm an acupuncturist can do is to puncture a lung if the needle goes deep enough. Other than that the possibility of anything else going wrong was rare if not unheard of. Well something, alas, did go terribly wrong and because of what happened I really do think I am unique in all the history of acupuncture. I am convinced of it.

Since I was still on the cube, I decided to telephone the Institute and ask for their advice about my having acupuncture for tinnitus. "We don't recommend it," Stephen said, "because acupuncture suppresses the illness whereas we bring it out. We have to go back over it."

"Which overrides the other?" I asked.

"Acupuncture," he said. Then added, "If you are going to have acupuncture tell them about your stomach. They can cure it."

Immediately I set about finding a suitable acupuncturist. It didn't prove difficult.

In the local press I saw an advert for an acupuncturist who was also a qualified doctor. He didn't live far away and I would be able to drive myself there and back easily in the car. The doctor answered the telephone and I asked firstly if there was anything he could do about my allergies. He wasn't too optimistic about helping me on that issue, but when I mentioned my tinnitus he said, "That's a different case altogether. I have been successful with tinnitus."

An appointment was made for the following day.

He turned out to be a very talkative Scottish gentleman who had just moved to London with his wife to be near his children. Concerning tinnitus he said, "I have a patient who is an old man of 90. He has had tinnitus since the First World War and he's deaf. Unfortunately, I wasn't able to cure him. He comes for treatment every three months—when it re-occurs."

Probably because he was a medical doctor he set about asking me numerous questions regarding the state of my health and I told him everything. "It all began with my eye infection," I said, "I took antibiotics for over three months, which resulted in my having the yeast fungus infection called Candida." He nodded as if he understood and I went on, "My whole body was affected. I had sickness and diarrhoea, allergies, continual throat infections, palpitations and so-called 'panic attacks' and aches and pains all over my body—practically everything. And because my immune system was so depleted I caught a severe virus which resulted in my having a vibration and a high-pitched sound in my right ear."

I went on to tell him about my visit to Dr Hibberd and the anti-Candida diet I was following, plus the many supplements I was taking.

He seemed appalled by it all, saying, "You've suffered more than some people do in twenty years."

He took my pulses by placing three fingers on the wrist of first one hand and then the other on what is called the radial artery. It is the Chinese method of diagnosis I had read about beforehand: its strength, rhythm and quality indicate the balance of energy and the state of disease. There is also the tongue diagnosis, but he didn't ask to see my tongue. The tongue, through its shape, colour, movement and coating indicates the progression and degree of the illness. The vital energy of the body is Ch'i (pronounced chee) but it is unknown in Western medicine. It keeps the blood circulating, warms the body and fights disease and it flows through certain channels forming a network within the entire body and linking all parts and functions together so that they work as one unit.

Acupuncture is a method of using fine needles to stimulate these invisible lines of energy running beneath the surface of the skin. It affects a change in the energy balance of the body and works to restore health.

-280As the doctor put needles around my ears he said, "The stone age men pierced themselves with primitive weapons and gradually they noticed that being pierced on certain parts of their body made their illnesses disappear."

Whilst I sat there with the needles in he showed me a book on acupuncture. It stated that tinnitus responds very well to acupuncture, which was very encouraging.

I sat there for about twenty minutes and he went on to chat about his family and how as a doctor he came to study acupuncture.

"I wanted to relieve pain," he said simply. 'That's the reason why most of my patients come to me."

He didn't say where he received his training and so I assumed he was self-taught.

"I want to see you in a few day's time and then once weekly for a time. I can't guarantee anything, but there should be an improvement after the fourth treatment," he said.

I told my neighbour that I was having acupuncture treatment for tinnitus and she became very interested. She suffered from high blood pressure and Raynauds disease, which causes circulation problems. She had been told to give up smoking but had so far failed to do so, "If I don't smoke I cry all day," she said. The GP, Miss Knight, the lady who had dismissed my Candida illness as nonsensical, had told her that there was no point in referring her to a specialist whilst she continued to smoke. "If you must go around with a dummy in your mouth all day..." was how she put it, which naturally had upset my neighbour greatly.

The second time I went for treatment she came along with me and the doctor gave her treatment to help her stop smoking.

A week later, after my third treatment, I woke up one morning to find that there was no ringing or vibration in my ear. I was absolutely overjoyed, but, sadly, after I began to move about it came back.

I told the doctor on my next visit about what happened and he said, "There was a reason for that. It didn't happen on its own," which gave me the determination to carry on.

During that time the lady of the newly formed tinnitus group wrote to me telling me where and when the meeting was to be held, which was in a centre close to home.

About five or six people turned up. They were all elderly and all of them had, along with their tinnitus, hearing difficulties. I felt totally out of place. A nurse had come to talk to us about our affliction but she annoyed me by saying, "Your hearing defect has caused your tinnitus."

Immediately I retorted, "But they told me that my hearing was perfect."

"Oh it only has to degenerate the tiniest bit," she replied, dismissing me completely. All she seemed interested in was obtaining hearing aids for the rest of the group and telling them that Dr Jonathan Hazel now did cochlea implants, which, I am sure, was good news to them, but it didn't help me in the least and I decided I wouldn't go again, even though, in the New Year, they intended inviting speakers who would give the group the latest information on the research that was being carried out regarding tinnitus and also help with the management of it.

Tinnitus, I knew, was not an illness itself but a symptom of something that had gone wrong.

It was then that something fateful happened to me. It came about because my neighbour, the one I had taken along with me to see the doctor about her smoking problem, gave me the name and telephone number of an acupuncturist who had a Chinese acupuncture clinic in the West End. Apparently he had helped a friend of hers. I telephoned him to find out if he had had any success with tinnitus, not intending to have treatment with him.

"How long have you had it?" he asked.

"Five months," I replied.

"That's good," he said, buoyantly. "If you had said five years then that would have been a different matter. I can guarantee, if not a cure, a 70% improvement."

"I've had four treatments with another acupuncturist. Does it matter?" I asked.

"No," he replied. "Did it get worse?"

"No," I told him.

"Then it should have," he retorted.

Because he seemed so confident that he could help me I made an appointment to see him the very next day. I realise now that it was an absolutely foolish thing to do to change acupuncturists. I hadn't given the doctor/acupuncturist a chance, but such was my anxiety and state of mind at the time. I was clutching at straws and I felt a Chinese acupuncturist would be more skilful.

The acupuncturist was from Taiwan and his clinic in the West End turned out to be very dismal. Nevertheless, I was not put off and, ironically, the first words I said to him were, "You won't upset the apple cart will you?"

He shook his head.

"How often have you been having treatment?" he enquired.

"Once a week," I replied.

Immediately he burst out laughing. "Western man does not understand the concept of acupuncture," he said. "You can come here three or four times a week at first...and then you can lessen it off. Come for twelve sessions and we will aim for a 70% improvement. Then you can come every three months for a booster, is that all right?"

"I want a cure," I said emphatically.

"Well it's very good," he replied. "You've only had it for five months."

"Have you ever had any cures?" I enquired.

"Well they never come back," he said, with satisfaction, "but I had one man who was too lazy to finish his treatment. When it was better he didn't bother to come, and when the ringing started again he would come again for treatment, but I couldn't help him. There was nothing I could do for him. He had had tinnitus in both ears for twenty years."

I was asked to sit down and he began to take my pulses.

"You're in a very weakened state," he said.

That was certainly true. The Candida problem had taken its toll and the cube had had a further devastating effect on my body. I was almost two weak to walk.

"Your small intestine is very weak," he went on. I just nodded. It was acupuncture jargon which I didn't understand.

The room was indeed dingy. The curtains were closed and there was a naked bulb in the centre. I was then asked to lie on the bed and he placed needles around both ears and on my hands and feet.

I asked him why he put them in my hands and feet and he replied, "It's the meridian up to the ears."

"Will it get worse?" I asked.

"It will get worse for the first couple of treatments, but then begin to get better," he replied. "The eyes and ears are the most difficult to treat. Sinus trouble for instance…it's gone after one treatment."

He left me to attend to other patients in adjoining rooms and I lay there for 45 minutes trying to relax as best I could, not knowing what terrible consequences my actions would bring.

At the end of the session I made a couple of appointments for the following week and paid him for twelve sessions in advance because he said it was cheaper that way.

That Sunday, I happened to attend the local Spiritualist Church that I continued to go to from time to time. That night there was a gentleman medium that seemed to be very accurate. He was coming to the end of his evening of clairvoyance when suddenly he pointed to me. "I would like to speak to that lady," he said.

Immediately I became too choked to answer, so I just nodded.

"You've been through hell, mentally and physically," he went on.

Tears welled up into my eyes and again I just nodded. He was so uncannily accurate. He paused for a moment and then he suddenly became extremely agitated. "Just stand back and view the situation," he said hastily. "Don't rush around trying everything—you might make a mistake!"

I didn't know how I could possibly make a mistake but it was clearly a warning. Little did I know that I was already in the process of making that mistake.

Then after a lengthy pause the medium suddenly said, "Oh I'm not going on. I've said too much already." The meeting ended at that point, but as the medium left the platform I walked up to him and, recognizing me as the lady he had just spoken to, he said, "Some people have to suffer a lot during their lifetime…but I promise that you won't always have to suffer."

Around that time I made an appointment to see Irene and Gerald Sowter at their healing centre in Reigate. I had to wait a couple of weeks because, as usual, they were so busy. Gerald Sowter had told me that they had had success with tinnitus and everything was worth a try.

"How long did it take?" I asked him.

"How long is a piece of string?" he replied.

Meanwhile, I continued to see the Taiwan acupuncturist and on the third and fourth occasions I went to the clinic he had electrical equipment alongside the bed.

"Look," he said. "I've got it all ready for you. You're a big girl now."

I lay on the bed and he inserted the needles around my ears and on various points on my arms and legs. Electrodes were attached to each needle. That was to stimulate them. The Chinese used to stimulate each needle by hand. Maybe they still do, but it is a very lengthy process. I went along with everything he did because he seemed to have absolute confidence in himself.

On the two occasions I lay on the bed for almost an hour while the needles around my ears and on my arms and legs vibrated away. But to my dismay, after the second time, my head didn't stop vibrating, the ringing in my ear was more pronounced and my ear began to vibrate frantically. I became very alarmed and when next I saw him I told him that everything was much worse.

"I'm not worried," he said impatiently, "and I'm treating you." He revealed his apprehension then because he added, "But you've had the harsh treatment, now we will bring it down."

He didn't put electrodes on the needles again but things continued to get worse.

I saw him a few times the following week and J kept asking him how long it would be before things improved. He just evaded the question.

Then, to my horror, I began to feel an odd sensation in my head. It seemed to be swimming in something and the whole of the top of my head seemed to be vibrating.

When next I saw him I pressed him to tell me what was happening to me.

"The Ch'i is remaining in the head," he said. "But once it gets through...."

"But when will it go?" I asked him, becoming more and more frantic.

"Three days...a month...two months and then gone," he said, clapping his hands.

What he said and the way he behaved seemed to me to be totally irresponsible. He had filled my head full of Ch'i or energy and it was a force that I could actually feel. It was very frightening and, needless to say, I never went to his clinic again.

I had seen an osteopath a couple of times previous to that and when I telephoned liim and told him what had happened he said, "Get in touch with the Scottish acupuncturist immediately," which I did.

"Please will you give me an appointment right away. It's urgent," I said, almost hysterically.

I don't know what he must have thought but he agreed to see me that afternoon and when the time came I drove myself to his house in a complete state of panic.

I told him frantically that I had seen another acupuncturist and had ten treatments in three weeks.

"You had ten treatments in three weeks!" he said incredulously. "I would have taken ten weeks."

"And he put electrical stimulation on my head and body for an hour on two consecutive days," I went on, "and after the second time my head didn't stop shaking and all the Ch'i has gone into my head."

"Well electrical stimulation is supposed to calm things down," he replied simply.

"He said I was a big girl now," I babbled on.

"Well I don't know what being a big girl has to do with it," he replied, "but some treatments are harsh...it's like bursting a bubble...but it obviously didn't work in your case. Well, we'll see if we can get back to where we left off. But what's the point if you go rushing off to somebody else again?" I assured him that I wouldn't do that again, but I sensed that he had lost interest in me because I had so foolishly left him to go elsewhere, which he had every right to do. But what was more worrying was the fact that he didn't seem to understand the full implication of what had happened.

He shook his head and said, "I have never had any trouble with acupuncture," and proceeded to put needles in my head and around my ears which I knew, even then, was totally the wrong treatment.

After the treatment, however, because I was in such a state, he even tried to hypnotise me in an effort to calm me down.

Alas it didn't work and I left in an even more hysterical state.

I was again all alone in the most appalling state, with something I didn't understand. My ear continued to ring and vibrate frantically at that time but what was going on in my head was another matter. It was horrendous. I used to feel something rising in my head which would then sizzle all over the top of my head making a loud noise and it seemed as if sparks were flying all over my face. The Ch'i bore into the top of my head and I felt as if I was going mad. I had never heard or read of such a thing happening before. That is why I feel I am unique in this matter. I doubt whether anyone has had his or her head full of Ch'i before. But thank God some acupuncturists believed what I told them and gave me treatment to channel it away from my head and they happened to be the top in their field in this country. The lesser ones dismissed me as a crank and the conventional doctors, of course, didn't believe me.

During the time I was receiving treatment from the Taiwan acupuncturist, I received a letter from the Institute telling me that they didn't recommend acupuncture whilst being on the cube! But, alas, the warning was not anywhere near strong enough, and anyway it had come too late. But whether the fact that I was still on the cube when I received the treatment had anything to do with what happened I really don't know and probably never will.

But immediately I was aware that something had gone terribly wrong. I telephoned the Institute, told them what had happened and asked to be taken off the cube, which they did immediately.

Not knowing where to turn I telephoned the Taiwan acupuncturist and told him exactly what I was experiencing in the head.

"The treatment was too harsh," I said, "and you shouldn't have put electrical stimulation on my head."

"That won't hurt you," he replied impatiently. "But it should have gone in a few days."

Well it hadn't gone in a few days, and when my husband telephoned him to ask what answer he had to the appalling situation I was in he said, "Take her to a specialist and have her head examined. She's got a blockage somewhere!"

In my desperation I began telephoning acupuncturists at random which turned out to be a very unwise thing to do. Most said that they had never had any trouble with acupuncture when I told them what had happened and refused to believe that I could actually feel excess Ch'i in the head, whilst one gentleman just said, "Look, I'm very busy," and slammed down the receiver, thinking probably that some nut case was telephoning him. But one acupuncturist asked me who had been responsible for putting the Ch'i in my head and when I told him he said, after a moment or two, "He's not on any lists. You could sue him. He's turned you upside down and it's irreversible. Personally, I wouldn't treat you because if I left you in a worse state you could sue me."

I didn't think how I could possibly be in a worse state but what he said frightened me—that it was irreversible!

Later in the evening, I was so distraught that I telephoned the number again. His wife answered.

"Don't you think that it was irresponsible of your husband to tell me that it was irreversible?" I said.

"Well, he's only speaking the truth'" she replied coldly.

"But I could have committed suicide," I said.

"Well that's up to you," she replied and slammed down the receiver.

After that episode I stopped telephoning acupuncturists at random. Not knowing where to turn, I simply telephoned Neal's Yard and asked to see a herbalist. I don't know why. I suppose it was to be.

"Beatrice is very good," the receptionist replied, "but she won't be here until next week."

I made an appointment for the following week.

Meanwhile, desperately wanting to contact the medium whose warning had been so accurate only weeks before, I telephoned the Spiritualist Church and spoke to the chairman. I asked him if I could have the telephone number of the medium concerned but he said, "As it happens he telephoned today, but he doesn't give private interviews so there's no point in my giving you his number. But I have the telephone number of another medium who has been here. I went to her flat for a reading. She's very good."

I wrote down the name and telephone number of the medium and thanked him.

The medium's name was Dawn Quayle. I hadn't heard of her but I couldn't wait to telephone for an appointment and I did so the same day. A soft female voice answered.

"Could you give me an appointment as soon as possible?" I asked. And I went on, "I'm in a desperate state. But I'm not interested in receiving messages from the dead. I just want clairvoyance."

"Well perhaps you had better go to a fortune teller," she replied sweetly.

"Well can you see the future?" I asked impatiently.

"Oh yes," she again replied sweetly. But she must have sensed my distress because she went on, "I think you had better come to the flat at 6 p.m. this evening and I will give you a reading. I will have put little John to bed by then. I have a child of two years old."

"Very well," I said. "I will definitely come."

She gave me her address and although I knew it was somewhere in the vicinity, because of the telephone number, I was delighted to find out that she lived only a short walking distance from my home, in a block of flats facing the main road.

I went along to the flat at six o'clock and John, her husband, opened the door.

Dawn turned out to be a very pretty lady with long golden hair. She looked in her twenties and I remarked, "You look very young to be a medium."

"Oh," she replied, with a smile, "I've been seeing spirits since I was five years old."

The flat was very tiny but cosy.

"Sit down on the settee and John will bring you a nice cup of tea," she said.

I made myself comfortable on the settee and John put a cassette into the tape recorder. Then he went to make a cup of tea, which he handed to me soon afterwards.

Meanwhile, Dawn had begun her reading.

"Darling you're going to get better," she said excitedly.

"Don't tell me that if it's not true," I implored.

"No, I wouldn't say that if it wasn't true…I would say it's going to be a slow process, but my guide says, 'She's going to be OK'," she said. She paused and then went on, "Were you going to take an overdose, because I can see a lot of tablets."

I shrugged my shoulders. "God only knows what is going to happen," I muttered to myself.

"Don't do it," she said. "Shall I tell you why? If you take your own life it is going against the laws of spirit and you are in complete despair and darkness and you won't know where to turn. You will keep on the earth plane. It takes a long time, besides there is no need. Have you seen Tom Johannson?"

'No," I replied, "but I am going to see a healer in Reigate—a lady who gives spirit operations. I've tried to see Tom Johannson but they won't even put me on a waiting list," I replied.

"He is in charge of all the mediums who work at the SAGB and he heals there himself on certain Saturday mornings," she said. "I work at the SAGB and I know Tom Johannson, I'll arrange an appointment for you, just tell them at the reception desk that you are Dawn Quayle's aunt. Go along this Saturday morning."

I told her how grateful I was and she went on with the reading saying, "You need mental rest, try and calm yourself down, because all will be well. The number of times the spirits tell me what to do and I've ignored it."

I promised to try and calm down.

"Have you recently been trying herbal remedies? I can see all herbal remedies around you," she went on.

"I have been taking herbs and I'm going to see a herbalist next week," I replied.

"You're getting healing from spirit," she continued, "but it's not easy. What I am picking up at the moment is a lot of confusion. I can't seem to be doing anything without confusion."

"I don't know where to turn," I said tearfully.

"I'm getting that you've got a long time on the earth plane and I can see a lot of happiness around you," she went on.

I must have looked somewhat sceptical because she added, "It's more than my job is worth to tell you things if you don't believe me."

"I'm afraid it will never go," I said in despair.

"It will go, have faith," she said, and she went on, "I can see you in the summer time laughing with a crowd of people around you. It's a good sign, hold on to it." What she said was indeed reassuring and she went on, "I can see a lot of paper around you. Who's writing?"

"That's me," I said at once.

"I can see a book on your lap," she said. "It will be finished by the end of the year 1989. I'm not saying it will be published by then but it will be finished."

I was only living from day to day at that time and two years seemed an eternity away to me.

"What does America mean to you?" she asked before ending her reading.

"Nothing," I replied, "except that I would like to go again."

"You will go again," she said with a smile.

I paid her fee and before I left she said, "Go along to see Tom Johannson on Saturday morning. Be early because it's first come first served, and go along to see the lady who gives spirit operations. Come here every evening at 6 o'clock and John will give you healing."

I promised to do that and indeed I went to the flat on numerous occasions for healing. Sometimes Dawn would give me healing and then John would massage my neck and back to try and relax the muscles. But there were times when I was in such torment that I wasn't able to go there.

When Saturday came my husband drove me to the SAGB in Belgrave Square. I arrived there at 9.30 a.m., being the first to arrive, and I waited half an hour outside before the doors were opened, but I didn't mind. Dawn had told me to be early. Another gentleman had arrived early and whilst we both stood waiting in the cold I asked if he had seen Tom Johannson.

'No," he replied, "but I've been coming here regularly for two years. I wasn't able to walk when I first came but now, as you can see, I can walk quite well."

He obviously had great faith in spiritual healing.

The attendant opened the doors punctually at 10 a.m.

"I'm Dawn Quayle's aunt," I said to him and, without hesitation, he nodded his head and said, "Go down to the large room at the end of the corridor." He pointed in the direction.

All alone in the room I sat patiently waiting for Tom Johannson to arrive. A little later a couple came in and sat down, but, because he was such a famous healer, I had expected crowds of people waiting to see him, especially since I was being told by those at the SAGB that it was pointless being put on the waiting list.

Tom Johannson eventually came into the waiting room. He was older than I had expected and was obviously taken aback when I stood up to introduce myself, having never seen me before, and, by the way he looked at me, I thought for a moment he was going to refuse to see me, but he took me into the chapel on the ground floor.

I sat down on a chair and at once convulsed into uncontrollable sobbing, and through my sobs I tried to explain to him what an appalling state I was in.

He placed his hands firstly on my head and then on my shoulders. I knew he had had numerous cases of instant cures during his mass demonstrations, but somehow I knew I wouldn't be that fortunate. Everything has to be right for that to happen.

"It's all nerves," he said, whilst healing me. "Your thyroid gland is overworking, causing adrenaline to flow which disrupts the blood flow. You must sit down and meditate. Think of your legs getting more and more relaxed and then your whole body. It's up to you when you are healed."

If it's up to me then I will never be healed I thought, knowing I had no control over what had happened to me.

He laid his hands on me for about ten minutes and then sat down. He said, "I won't be here for the next couple of weeks but I'll tell Angela, my assistant, to see you. I'm training her. She's a very good healer. Unfortunately she's very unreliable, she comes when she feels like it, but I'll tell her you will be here at 11 a.m. next Saturday. I'll be here in three week's time and as from now you are on our absent healing list."

Dawn was very pleased when I told her that Tom Johannson had given me healing. Alas, the following Saturday, I turned up for my appointment with Angela, but there was no sign of her, which was very disappointing.

A few days after seeing Tom Johannson, I managed to drive myself to Reigate to see the healers Irene and Gerald Sowter.

Christmas was a few weeks away but the waiting room and chapel were already decorated with coloured lights and trimmings. Soft music was playing. The waiting area was, as usual, crowded, and as I sat there waiting to be seen tears poured down my cheeks. I despaired at the wretched and truly appalling situation I was in. Since I had been taken off the cube the intense aching had abated, but I still had some aches and pains and I still had the occasional stomach upset, but I no longer suffered from diarrhoea.

The Candida was easing thanks to the nystatin and Superdophilus plus all the supplements I continued to take. But there appeared no answer to the torment in my head.

Irene Sowter came into the waiting room and said, "I won't keep you long. I've had twenty four already this afternoon." But I wasn't in the least concerned at the length of time I had to wait.

Soon, however, Gerald came and took me into the healing centre. He asked me to lie on one of the beds and a lady assistant proceeded to give me healing whilst I waited to be seen by Irene, who was attending to a patient in an adjoining room. Only a curtain partitioned it and I could hear everything that was going on.

"I'm going to give you a spirit operation," I heard Irene say.

The lady had come for the removal of a cataract. I had spoken to her previously in the waiting room and she had said, "I knew a person who had spiritual healing for cataracts and when the cataract was removed her eyesight was perfect." She was therefore filled with optimism.

Irene then breathed very heavily and after quickly going into a trance, she began to speak in a deep, gruff voice. It was the voice of her spirit doctor. It sounded so weird that it sent shivers down my spine. Nevertheless, I found it fascinating. I had never experienced anything like it before. I couldn't make out everything she said but it seemed her spirit doctor was giving her instructions as to what to do.

"Come back next week," she said to the woman at the end, speaking then in her normal voice.

Afterwards it was my turn and Irene came and stood by my bed, "I recognise you from the last time you came here," she said, before rushing off to find my file. When she returned she said, "You had stomach and bowel problems."

"Yes," I replied, "I had Candida—a yeast fungus infection."

She looked surprised, remembering, possibly, that all she had said to me was "Keep off the chips".

"What's the trouble now?" she asked, and I told her about the ringing in my ears and the Ch'i in my head.

"Ringing in the ears is a sign from the spirit world that they want to contact you," she said. It was complete rubbish as far as I was concerned, but I kept quiet not wishing to offend her.

"You want it removed?" she asked.

I nodded.

"Are you sure?" she asked.

"Absolutely sure!" I replied.

She then placed her hands on my head and said, "I can feel a lot of juggling." I knew what she meant—my head was full of Ch'i and her sensitive hands had picked it up. She then placed her hands on my body and said quickly, "You want to pass on." I nodded. It was true. I didn't know how long I could cope with the present torment that was in my head. "You'll be sorry," she whispered. Dawn had said the same thing but I hadn't ruled out the possibility of being forced to take my life. "The spirits are telling me that you must play the piano," she said. It stunned me because she had no idea that music was my great love—it is after all the food of the soul. I had a diploma in pianoforte playing and most of my youth had been taken up by practising the piano. I loved it.

"I'm going to give you a spirit operation," she said, and I lay on the bed whilst she began breathing very deeply and, quickly going into a trance, she began to speak in the low, gruff voice I had heard earlier.

For about ten minutes she poked her fingers in my right ear, wetting it and doing all sorts of funny things. At the end, when she was out of her trance, I asked her what she had been doing. "The spirits were relieving the congestion," she replied.

I made an appointment for the following week, but because I was in so much torment I wasn't able to go. In fact a day or two after seeing her I was in so much torment that I called for a minicab and went to the Emergency Department of King's College Hospital.

I told the minicab driver what had happened to me and he remarked, "I have never heard of acupuncture going wrong before!"

I was examined by a lady doctor who was clearly disturbed when I told her what I was experiencing in my head. She arranged for me to see an ENT specialist that afternoon. I went home again by minicab and returned with my husband in time for the afternoon session.

I was obliged to wait a long time before being seen by the doctor and I didn't think I would be able to stay the course. I walked up and down with the Ch'i sizzling away, making a considerable noise and boring into my head.

At last the time came for me to see the young specialist. He looked into both ears and said, "I can't find anything wrong with your ears. There are many causes for tinnitus." But when I told him what I was experiencing inside my head after having acupuncture treatment for tinnitus he too seemed alarmed. "Tell your doctor to send you to an acupuncturist. You can get one on the National Health," he said, "I can't do anything for you."

"You're sending me to my death," I said somewhat melodramatically. But it was true. I had no one to turn to for help. I knew the only way they could help me was to render me unconscious and they couldn't do that.

Anyway, I only had to wake up again and face the same situation—which was hell! And I remembered the words of the spirit voice, "what I can see for you". Was this what the spirit had seen?

After leaving the hospital I returned home, and as usual I did my best to get through the evening and night. I had no sleeping pills to help me at that time. Later, however, I was able to obtain a regular supply, which probably saved my life because when I found the torment too much for me to bear I was at least able to put myself to sleep. The sleeping pills were not obtained from my GP.

As the specialist had recommended, I went to see my GP, seeing the only member of the panel I hadn't seen before, a Miss Stevens (not her correct name). I deliberately avoided seeing the other two, regarding them as being totally useless.

She was a lady with definite views that, alas, were hopelessly different to mine. I told her what the specialist had said to me and she said, "I've never heard of acupuncture on the National Health Service."

But when I told her the reason for my request she snapped, "I don't believe in Ch'i," and she got up from her seat and opened the door and I was obliged to leave the surgery. To her, I was talking absolute nonsense.

The day of my appointment with Beatrice arrived and I went to Neal's Yard. She was young, pretty, with long dark hair. By that time the vibration and ringing had gone from my ear. The vibration had firstly moved to the top of my ear and then disappeared completely, presumably into the head. Everything had been pushed into my head. I told her the extent of my suffering and said, "It was caused by an acupuncturist after receiving treatment for tinnitus."

"I have never known anyone with such severe symptoms in the head," she replied, somewhat aghast and she went on, "I'm giving you a herbal mixture for congestion, but I'm very concerned at what you are experiencing. My husband is an acupuncturist and I'll talk to him about your case. Give me your telephone number." I quickly wrote it down on a piece of paper and handed it to her.

"Give me a ring in a few day's time," she said, and gave me, in return, her own private number.

I waited for a day or two before telephoning the number. Beatrice answered. "Have you spoken to your husband yet?" I asked eagerly.

"Yes," she replied, "I've discussed your case with him and he would like to speak to you."

Her husband came to the telephone.

"Yes," he said, "Beatrice has spoken to me about you and I've got in touch with another acupuncturist and discussed your case with him. You've got Ch'i in the head. Whatever you do don't have any more needles put into your head. Go to Giovanni Maciocia, I was a pupil of his, he's brilliant. He's an Italian and he has a western approach to acupuncture. I'll give you his telephone number."

I quickly wrote it down.

"Will it go on its own?" I asked hopefully.

"Yes," he answered, "but do you want to wait that long?"

I thanked him for his help. Little did I know that I would have to wait many years before it finally left my head. I telephoned Giovanni as soon as possible. He listened patiently when I told him everything that had happened.

"You must have needles put into the soles of your feet to bring the Ch'i down. It won't go after one treatment. You'll need treatment every day for a week," he said.

He was only in London for two mornings a week and was usually booked up well in advance, but he gave me an appointment for the following week.

Meanwhile, he gave me the names and telephone numbers of two of his colleagues, Felicity and Tina. "They will know what to do," he said. However, because there was now no ringing or vibration in the ear I cancelled my appointment with Dr Jonathan Hazel. It was now pointless.

CHAPTER 10

As soon as I had been given the telephone numbers of the two acupuncturists recommended by Giovanni I set about contacting them. I telephoned Felicity first and a lady with a strong Australian accent answered. I told her that Giovanni had given me her name and telephone number and what the problem was.

"Since it's an emergency you can come on Sunday at 1 p.m." she said. Sunday was the following day and I readily agreed.

Felicity turned out to be a very outgoing, friendly person. She wrote down all my symptoms and asked what treatment I had received from the Taiwan acupuncturist. To my surprise she said, "The treatment he gave you was all in order." She took my pulses and then said, "Undress to your pants and lie face down on the bed."

When I had done so she inserted needles in the soles of my feet and a few down my spine. She left me in the room for a while and then returned to take out the needles saying, "As soon as you arrive home I want you to lie down for about half an hour."

I quickly dressed and my husband drove me straight home. I did as I was told and lay down for half an hour, but when I got up it was as if a gale force wind rushed up from my spine into my neck and was shattering my ears. I had never experienced anything like that before and it was all very frightening.

I then telephoned Tina as soon as I could and found that she gave treatment at a flat in Pimlico which was a more convenient place for me to travel to. I made an appointment for a few days' time.

I went there by mini-cab and I arrived early. The tenant of the flat on the ground floor opened the door. Tina practised in the flat on the top floor.

"Strange and weird things go on up there," she said, which amused me.

Tina soon arrived and led me upstairs. She was a gently spoken young lady from South Africa. She listened carefully to all I had to tell her saying afterwards, "You've got too much Ch'i in the head," and she then added sympathetically, "I don't like to see people suffering," seemingly genuinely concerned about the plight I was in. "Take your tights off and lie face upwards on the bed," I was told. When I did so she inserted needles in the soles of my feet and in my hands saying, "You must have this kind of treatment. It will bring down the Ch'i. Each treatment is like laying a brick on top of a brick—it builds up."

"What went wrong with the treatment the Taiwan acupuncturist gave me?" I asked.

"You don't put electrical stimulation on the head for an hour on two consecutive days," she said. "I hardly ever use electricity…only in cases of extreme pain."

"But will it go?" I enquired anxiously.

"Yes it will go," she assured me.

I told her about the conversation I had had with the acupuncturist who had said that it was irreversible.

"You shouldn't be phoning up people at random," she replied, rather crossly. I had a few treatments with her before I saw Giovanni. She advised me to see a cranial osteopath in Clapham and I did have a number of treatments with her. She said she was adjusting the spinal fluid.

I went to Harley House to receive treatment from Giovanni Maciocia and he didn't seem to mind that I had already had a few treatments with Tina. He had studied acupuncture in China and was qualified to practise Chinese Traditional Medicine, being also qualified in Medical Herbalism, and he was thought to be the top acupuncturist in the country. Everyone I spoke to who knew anything about acupuncture had nothing but glowing words for him.

He took my pulses by placing his hand on the radial artery of both of my wrists and then asked to see my tongue. "The treatment you received was wrong," he said. "Your stomach and spleen are weak and by giving the head electrical stimulation it further depleted the stomach. The treatment was too strong for you."

I told him about the gale force wind I felt going up the back of my neck. He looked concerned and said, "You've got wind in the head, as the Chinese say."

I took off my tights and lay on the bed and he began puffing needles in my arms and legs and in my stomach.

"My tongue is not right is it?" I said, because it was still dry and red.

"It's not the tongue but the coating that tells us what is wrong," he said. "You've got too much mucous in the stomach." I nodded. It made sense.

"Acupuncture can't cause you any harm, except if you puncture a lung," he said confidently. But that to me was absolute nonsense. I was suffering the torments of hell because of a treatment, which, for some reason or other, went dreadfully wrong. After about twenty minutes he removed the needles and I put on my tights while he wrote out a prescription for me all in Chinese. "I've given you herbs for the wind in your head and herbs to bring down the Ch'i. There is a little Chinese herbalist in Soho. Take the prescription there and they will give you the necessary herbs," he said.

Before leaving, however, he had a word with my husband. "She has Ch'i in the head," he said, "but it won't do her any harm—it's only a force!"

At the Chinese herbalist I was given five packets of herbs. Each packet contained what looked like the bark of a tree. They had to be boiled in a pint of water and then simmered down to a cupful and then strained. It smelled foul and tasted even worse, but I persevered with it.

The night after my treatment with Giovanni, however, I woke up with the most terrible sensations in my head.

It seemed his treatment had had an effect on the Ch'i and I arose the following morning to find myself shaking from head to foot, which lasted all day.

Before seeing Giovanni again I had a few treatments with Tina who was pleased that I had been given a prescription for herbs but warned, "You shouldn't change treatments." It meant nothing to me at the time.

I again telephoned the Institute and told them exactly what had happened to me and that because I had had acupuncture whilst being on the cube I now had a head full of excess Ch'i. For a moment or two Mindi didn't answer, but she then said, "If you go back on the cube you will be more messed up!" I had no intention of going back on the cube-but it was too late, the damage had been done. What happened to me was cruel.

I managed to have a few more treatments with Giovanni before Christmas at Harley House and I even travelled to his home, miles away, to obtain treatment when he was not available in London. On that occasion he put moxibustion on my feet, which is the stimulation of energy by the use of burning herbs. The following day I shook even more violently from head to foot. Acupuncture, I now knew, was a very powerful form of treatment.

My husband usually drove me to Harley House, but one day before Christmas I went by mini-cab and I had the same driver who had driven me to King's College Hospital. He said, "I knew they wouldn't be able to do anything for you. The Ch'i has to be rechannelled."

During this terrible time Dawn and John were a great comfort to me. John gave me healing and Dawn would say repeatedly, "Don't worry, one day it will go."

I had gone to the SAGB every Saturday morning since I had received healing from Tom Johannson, but Angela had never turned up. I mentioned to Dawn that I hoped to see Tom Johannson again the following Saturday morning.

"I've left the SAGB," Dawn said. "I felt ill and didn't want to work, but Tom Johannson was so unreasonable that I just walked out."

"Oh," I gasped, "and I'm supposed to be your aunt."

"It won't make any difference," John said.

On the Saturday morning I arrived early at the SAGB and sat waiting to see Tom Johannson along with a young couple with two children who had arrived before me.

When he walked into the room, however, he completely ignored me and walked over to the young couple and greeted them cordially. They got up and walked out of the room and he followed. But before leaving the room, Tom Johannson stopped and glared at me. 'I haven't seen you before," he snapped icily, which so totally astounded me that I didn't answer. He went on to demand quite nastily, "Have you got an appointment?"

"I saw you a couple of weeks ago and you told me to come today. Don't you remember?" I managed to stumble out. "Meanwhile you said you would arrange for me to see Angela, but unfortunately she never turned up."

As soon as I began to speak, he swiftly turned his head away from me and said, "Oh that's different, you mean you want to see Angela."

"No, I want to see you," I pleaded. But he just turned his back on me and marched out of the room.

I sat there completely stunned. I couldn't believe that a man with such a wonderful gift of healing who was supposed to be so enlightened spiritually didn't even seem to know the meaning of the word charity.

Too shocked and disappointed by his behaviour to move, I continued to sit in the waiting room. Not long afterwards, another couple came into the waiting room. The lady wore a fabulous mink coat.

I was still sitting there when suddenly a very tall, smartly dressed black lady came bustling into the room. I guessed immediately it was Angela and when I asked her if she was, she said, "Yes, I'm Angela."

She agreed to give me healing and took me into one of the small rooms on the ground floor. But I couldn't help but tell her how badly Tom Johannson had behaved towards me and she said, "He deals mainly with rich foreigners who come over from the continent especially to see him. They give large donations to his hospitals in

Switzerland and Germany," which probably accounted for his appalling behaviour. It was obvious to me that he thought of me as expendable and the reason why I failed to get on the waiting list to see him was, in my opinion, because there was no waiting list as such.

Just before Christmas my husband and I were involved in a car crash. Nobody was hurt but we were both shaken up. The car was a complete write-off. It happened on a Saturday and on the Sunday morning I woke up with uncontrollable shaking. It was probably delayed reaction. But I was in such a bad state with the shaking and the sizzling in my head that I telephoned my GP.

Since it was a Sunday I had to telephone the emergency number. Miss Knight answered—the doctor who had refused to believe that I had Candida. I told her that I had been involved in a car accident and was shaking all over and with the sizzling in my head I felt suicidal.

"Have you ever tried to commit suicide before?" she asked nonchalantly.

"Yes. I've even counted the number of pills I'll need." I answered facetiously. I couldn't take her seriously.

"Well I think you had better go to a psychiatric hospital," she said with complete indifference.

"That won't do my head any good," I retorted and I went on to say, "but I've got a brilliant acupuncturist who is trying to get the Ch'i out of my head."

"Look," she said angrily, 'you're phoning me at half past twelve on a Sunday."

I couldn't believe what I was hearing. What the hell had the time of day got to do with it. I could have been dying for all she knew, so I retorted, "What are you doing…cooking the dinner? You're nothing but a stupid bitch."

That did it, she immediately slammed down the receiver, cutting off all contact, which to me was another stupid thing to do so I telephoned again, and when she knew that it was me she said, "I'm not going to be spoken to like that." But then added, "Come to the surgery tomorrow morning."

"What for?" I asked. "How can you possibly help me?"

"You'll see," she said, in her usual Irritating manner. Then adding sneeringly, "Or perhaps you would rather see your brilliant acupuncturist." I could have strangled her.

Nevertheless, I did go to the surgery the following morning, but I avoided seeing Miss Knight. I saw Miss Stevens instead. "We've looked through all your files and come to the conclusion that you must see a psychiatrist," she said sternly.

I had had enough of psychiatrists. They hadn't helped in the past and it wasn't the help I needed at that precise moment.

"I have an acupuncturist who is trying to bring down the Ch'i from my head," I said.

"I've told you that I don't believe in Ch'i," she snapped angrily. "We are back to the same thing again." And she angrily turned away from me indicating that that was the end of my time with her and once again I was obliged to get up and walk out of her room without further ado.

Every time I lay down there seemed to be more pressure in my head and the Ch'i was always worse, so I had difficulty in getting to sleep. On occasions I had to drink quite a considerable amount of whisky to make me relaxed enough to go to sleep.

I decided therefore to visit once again Miss Stevens and ask if I could be given some sleeping pills. "I can't be responsible for giving you sleeping pills. You might take too many," she retorted, and she began looking through my medical records saying, "I see that you've got funny feelings in the head and you are suicidal."

"That's rubbish," I snapped. "I'm not suicidal and I've got Ch'i in the head."

"Well that's what I've got down here," she replied sharply, "and I've already told you that I don't believe in Ch'i." And with that she got up from her seat and turned her back to me—once again informing me that my visit was over.

It was hopeless trying to talk sense to the two female doctors, so I decided to see the male doctor. I though he might prove more accommodating. Alas, he wasn't. All he wanted to do was to get me off the list. Knowing very well that I had been rude to one of his colleagues he said, "We work as a team here." In other words, what I had done to one I had done to the rest.

"Well, are you going to throw me off the list?" I questioned.

He didn't answer. But when I asked to be given sleeping pills because of the torment in my head he absolutely refused, saying, "We don't agree with them here!"

They didn't agree with sleeping pills! Their tunnel vision could have cost me my life. As I have already stated they proved my salvation. I don't know if I could have kept going without them.

Soon afterwards, I once again telephoned the Taiwan acupuncturist and told him the state I was m.

"Have you seen a specialist yet?" he asked.

"What for?" I replied. "It was the acupuncture that caused the trouble. You know I could sue you."

"Go ahead and try'" he sneered. "It's never happened before."

But with all his bravado he did seem worried about what had happened as well he should have been—it could have proved fatal.

"Are there any herbs that will bring down the Ch'i?" I asked, testing him to see whether he knew anything about herbs.

"Oh it's the Chinese New Year," he stammered, "and if there's one herb missing...." From that feeble attempt at an excuse I gathered that he knew nothing about herbs.

I didn't telephone him again, but after a year of absolute hell I wrote to him and told him that it was a miracle I was still alive.

Tina also practised at the Meridians and I went there on one or two occasions. On one occasion she was supervising two students—a man and a woman. The male student looked horrified when Tina said, "She had electrical stimulation on her head for an hour on two consecutive days and now she has too much Ch'i in the head. She says it sizzles, makes a noise and seems as if sparks are flying in her head and on her forehead."

"Can you see the sparks?" he asked.

"No, I can't see the sparks," I answered, somewhat impatiently.

Tina supervised while the lady student put in the needles, but she was so inexperienced they hurt and to her consternation I kept shouting out in pain.

After the treatment, however, for the rest of the night and the whole of the next day the Ch'i in my head seemed to go mad. I was unable to sleep so I paced the sitting room all night. Perhaps the treatment had been especially strong. The effects of a treatment had never lasted so long.

The following morning I telephoned Tina. "That's the way it goes sometimes," she replied nonchalantly.

But because the Ch'i didn't seem to be going significantly, even with treatment, I became so despondent that I asked Dawn to give me another reading. She readily gave me one even though she was always booked up well in advance.

"My guide says that you are going to get better, all will be well. She's saying to me, 'She will get better'. I can see you going over water—but I'm getting delays. It's not America but she's not telling me where." And she went on, "I think I've given you this before. I feel as if I'm in a cave—totally black, but there is a split in it and it's going to open…. in fact it has already opened. That's the only way I can explain it to you…. they are showing me symbolically. 'Her future…. she cannot see it…. she's completely enclosed in this dark cave…. but it's opening up…. it has already started.' As you sit there I can feel this heaviness around you. But all will be well."

"Is your guide sure all will be well?" I enquired despondently.

"Spirits never lie," she replied sweetly. "Try and relax and calm yourself."

On another occasion I went to the flat in a state of absolute torment, not knowing what to do with myself. Dawn held my hand and repeated, "My guide says that you will get better. It will go. She says you are better but not aware of it. She says you are in a simmering period." And she went on to whisper in my ear, "Noises in the head are worse than cancer. I had it for a year…every time I lay do…. and it was very loud. John cured me. I thought I was going mad—well I was mad. They put me in a straightjacket and locked me in a padded cell."

She certainly knew what suffering was all about. Perhaps that was why she could sympathise with and relate so well to the suffering of others. I knew that she had a background of abject poverty. "My father was an alcoholic," she once told me. But what I didn't know was the sad fact that she too was an alcoholic. I was to find out that fact a few months later.

Christmas came and went. During that time I had been unable to receive treatment. Meanwhile Giovanni had told me to massage my feet in an effort to bring do. the Ch'i.

It altered all the time. Sometimes it would seem as if it was boring a hole in my head while others it seemed to spread out all over the top of my head and sizzle, making a considerable noise.

I had a few treatments with Giovanni after Christmas. Tina had gone to South Africa for a short while. But my appointment time at Harley House was invariably at 9.30 a.m. which was very inconvenient. My husband had to take me there in the car and then dash off to work. I usually returned home by taxi. And I wasn't able to have regular treatment because being in London on only two mornings a week he was inundated with patients and he couldn't always fit me in. So I began to look for a clinic where I could obtain more regular treatment. I did so reluctantly because I knew Giovanni had a great reputation. And apart from him, Tina and Felicity, no other acupuncturist had taken me seriously.

I did see a black osteopath at that time who was also a trained acupuncturist but he refused to give me acupuncture treatment saying, "in China you only have twelve acupuncture treatments and then you are not allowed to have acupuncture again for a whole year."

I told him that I had received treatment from Giovanni but my head still seemed full of Ch'i.

"I met Giovanni when we were both students in Nanjing," he said. "I'm sure he's done his best for you," which was not at all encouraging.

CHAPTER 11

By February 1987 the Ch'i in my head had only gone down by a very small fraction and it still caused me considerable distress.

It was then that I noticed an advert for an acupuncture clinic in Ealing called The Liu clinic, run by a Dr Liu.

I telephoned the clinic one morning and spoke to a lady acupuncturist. It happened to be the morning that the Well Woman Clinic was being held. Dr Liu himself was not present. I told her that I had been receiving treatment from Mr Giovanni Maciocia and she said at once, "Well he's the top acupuncturist in the country."

"Yes, I know that," I replied, "but I'm finding it very difficult to have regular treatment with him, with one thing and another.

I went on to explain that the problem was too much Ch'i in the head but she appeared not to fully comprehend what I was saying. Anyway, she said that she would send me more information about the clinic and indeed within a few days I received a letter and more information regarding the clinic. In her letter she referred to the torment in my head as tinnitus and not as excess Ch'i, which is what I told her it was. Naturally it didn't please me, but in any case I would never have been able to get to the clinic on that one morning a week.

The clinic, I read in the pamphlets sent to me, was founded by Dr Liu in 1975 and it practised Traditional Chinese Medicine in its entirety. It was the first clinic in the West to admit in-patients as well as out-patients for intensive treatment and what was most interesting was the fact that it encouraged co-operation with practitioners of Western medicine and medical doctors were at hand to prescribe and administer Western medicine. Dr Liu was himself a medical doctor. The clinic offered many therapeutic methods of treatment, which included acupuncture, moxibustion, cupping, herbal medicine, meditation, massage and Tai Ch'i classes. 'The treatment of Traditional Chinese Medicine', it stated, 'comes from a long tradition of knowledge and experience'. Dr Liu, I was told later, came from a long line of acupuncturists. It all seemed so impressive that I felt compelled to telephone Dr Liu. When I did I told him that I had too much Ch'i in my head. To my surprise he didn't dispute the fact.

"If you've got too much Ch'i in the head then something is wrong. I've been treating patients for thirty years…it takes a long time to learn about acupuncture and there are a lot of cowboys about."

I was well aware of that fact.

I made an appointment for a consultation at his clinic a few days later. The clinic was open from 2 p.m. to 6 p.m. every weekday and on a Saturday morning, which meant that I could receive treatment when-ever I could get to the clinic, which was wonderful for me.

His clinic was in a detached house in Ealing. It was very clean and well run. Everyone at that time was worried about the possibility of catching AIDS from infected needles -they probably still are, but Dr Liu assured everyone that his needles were thoroughly sterilized before use, which they were, by placing them in a machine which generated great heat. When I went to Giovanni's house for treatment I noticed that he had a similar machine. Nowadays a lot of acupuncturists use disposable needles—they have to.

At my consultation with Dr Liu he asked me what exactly had hap-pened after the Taiwan acupuncturist had treated me. I told him what I was experiencing in my head.

"What does the acupuncturist say about it?" he asked, without asking his name.

"He said that I had a blockage in the head and the Ch'i couldn't get through," I told him.

He looked somewhat surprised, but then asked, "Well has the tinni-tus in the ear gone?"

I nodded.

"He's pushed it into the head. It has to be brought down," he concluded.

He then set about diagnosing my 'illness' by consulting the yi-sheng. He placed his hands on the radial artery of my wrists, thus taking my pulses. He noted down which were the strong or weak organs of the body so that the correct method of treatment could be selected.

Since I had travelled such a long distance by car asked if he would give me treatment straight away. He agreed and so I was asked to undress to my panties and lie on one of the beds. There were two rooms with four or five beds in each. Curtains partitioned off the beds. The place was centrally heated, which I was grateful for—it was the depths of winter.

Dr Liu began putting needles in me saying, "Have twenty treatments and then come back for a booster a month later. It will go."

He inserted about thirty needles altogether, some each side of my neck, which he said was where the problem lay, on my shoulders, down my spine and in my arms and legs. I had never had so many needles stuck into me. Each needle was then attached to an electrode to stimulate them and they all pulsated. But I had every confidence in him and I began attending the clinic two or three times a week. I always found him to be full of optimism, which he passed on to his patients. He knew the power of the mind and positive thinking. To him anything is possible—which I suppose it is.

I still had the occasional trouble with my stomach at that time and aches and pains all over my body and I would ask him to treat every problem as well as bringing down the Ch'i raging in my head and I would cry the whole time. Nobody ever understood the torment I was going through. It was such a unique case that I couldn't really expect people to understand. But Dr Liu never argued with the fact that I had too much Ch'i in my head. When he was needling my feet he would say, "You should be feeling tingling in the feet," which I didn't at that time but I did quite some time later when the Ch'i had been noticeably brought down.

During the time I attended the clinic I met some very brave and wonderful people. There was Maggie, a pretty young lady who was the only in-patient at the clinic at the time, and had a nurse to look after her.

"When she came first to the clinic she had several treatments a day, she was in so much pain," Stella, Dr Liu's assistant, told me.

It seems that Maggie had been filming a TV commercial that showed a couple pulling into the pit at Silverstone, mistaking it for a petrol station. Maggie was told to run across the track at the wrong time and was hit by a car and sent flying. She suffered a crushed pelvis and broken leg and was hospitalised for months. Shell paid her medical expenses although they had no liability in the matter. "They have been very good to me," she said.

When I first attended the clinic Maggie always seemed to be having treatment, but she didn't like the needles and I could hear her shout out in agony when Dr Liu inserted the needles 'inches deep' as she would say.

"We both have to be brave," she said to me, but I didn't want to have to be brave—all I begged for was to be out of my torment so that I could lead a normal life again.

A few months later she told me she was about to have a hip replacement operation, but when I stopped going to Dr Liu' 5 clinic I heard no more about her until I read in the Equity Journal of March 1989 that she had been awarded the highest damages ever for an Equity member and that she said she owed her life to the Consultant Orthopaedic Surgeon who had carried out the delicate hip replacement operation. I wish her well.

Also attending the clinic at that time was another brave lady. She had ME which is short for Myalgic Encephalomyelitus or Post Viral Syndrome.

"I had glandular fever," she told me, "and that's one of the viruses that don't leave you. I was so ill I was in bed for five months. I used to lie there and wait for it to get dark so that I could go to sleep."

-280"How does it affect you?" I enquired sympathetically.

"My muscles ache tremendously and I feel sick. I am too weak to walk, but I'm lucky not to be in a wheelchair. A lot of the other sufferers are in wheelchairs and their muscles are wasting."

"What does Dr Liu do for you?" I enquired.

"He keeps moving the Ch'i around. I don't want to get too low. I told my doctor that I was having acupuncture treatment but he just smiled. He doesn't believe in Ch'i."

"I know about that only too well," I told her. "I have the same problem."

She knew there was no cure in sight and that the illness could last up to twenty years, but she said hopefully, "My doctor is always on the alert for anything new that might come along."

Also attending the clinic was an old gentleman who walked with crutches. He was in such pain in his back that he couldn't walk. He had been advised to seek help at Dr Liu's clinic by a workman who came to do some work on his house. Seeing his plight he told him that his own wife had been considerably eased of her pain by Dr Liu. I spoke to the old gentleman and he said, "I was very miserable when I came here. I had seen all the specialists and they gave me painkiller after painkiller with the result that I had a huge jar full of codeine tablets. It was hopeless. But after five or six treatments with Dr Liu I'm now able to walk to the clinic with the aid of a stick only and I'm free of pain for the first time in years." The smile on his face showed it all. And he went on, "I've told my daughter about the relief I have experienced. She has MS and she is badly affected by the disease. She now attends the clinic."

Later I was to meet the lady on a number of occasions. She was a delightful woman, always pleasant and charming and so pretty. But after a number of treatments she was able to get around a lot better and one day she said to me, "Yesterday I was able to see my garden for the first time in years."

Another young man I met at the clinic had a rather amusing experience. "I could write a book about GPs," he said to me, and I muttered to myself, "You're not alone in that

so can we all." However, he went on, "The hospital took a year to find out what was wrong with me. I had lethargy so severe I couldn't work. My speech was affected and I couldn't concentrate. Eventually they found that I had thyroid gland malfunction. Then, one Christmas Eve, I noticed a rash on my lower abdomen, so I went to my GP. When I showed him my abdomen he threw his hands in the air and shouted in horror, 'Don't come near me, you've got secondary syphilis' so I simply said to him, 'Thank you doctor. On Christmas Eve too.' I got rid of the rash myself by using chamomile lotion. So much for my secondary syphilis!"

Around Easter time I had another cytotoxic test at the Laboratories in Putney. Believe it or not at that time I was still taking nystatin and Superdophilus plus the many supplements. But, of course, with all the torment in my head everything else was secondary. Nevertheless, I felt that I had at last overcome Candida and I wasn't surprised when the results came back to find that I was no longer reacting to any food or chemical. I suppose it was some consolation and I began reducing my dosage of nystatin, soon leaving it off altogether. But I continued to take Superdophilus for some time to come.

Unfortunately, around that time I caught a severe bladder infection and I was obliged to go to see one of the doctors on the panel. I saw Miss Stevens, the young lady who didn't believe in Ch'i. The first time I saw her she told me to take paracetemol for my intense backache—everything it seemed could be cured by paracetemol—but, because after almost a week there was no improvement, I went again to see her and this time she arranged for me to have a urine test. The sample went to St Thomas' Hospital. I telephoned the surgery a few days later and the receptionist told me that my urine was infected so I was obliged to call the doctor again. She gave me antibiotics to clear the infection, which I was loath to take, and told me to come back in a week's time bringing with me another urine sample that would be tested again to see if the infection had gone.

I had the most severe aching in my back and in my legs so I contacted Beatrice and she very kindly sent me a herbal medicine to ease my aching. But when next I saw Miss Stevens I mentioned that I had been taking a herbal remedy. She just glared at me and said crossly, "You can stop taking herbs. They won't do you any good."

I had given up mentioning that I still had Ch'i in my head and now she was telling me that she didn't believe in herbs either. It was ludicrous and it strengthens the idea that medical doctors should spend some time during their long training learning about alternative methods of healing.

CHAPTER 12

About 9 a.m. one morning, not long after Easter, I had a telephone call from John.

"Can you come to the flat immediately?" he said frantically. "Dawn's daughter has been killed in a road accident and she's in a terrible state. Two women have been with her the whole night. And would you bring a bottle of drink with you...anything."

I thought it was an unusual request but I agreed to bring a bottle with me. I went immediately to buy a bottle of vodka, thinking that Dawn probably needed something strong after hearing that tragic news.

When I arrived at the flat I found Dawn in a pitiful state, lying on the settee, eyes swollen with crying, but what shocked me was the fact that she was completely inebriated.

"That's the third child I've lost," she said, slurring her words, "a son and a daughter and a still birth."

I knew she had been married before but I didn't know she had had children.

Dawn then got up from the settee and started banging her head on the floor. I did my best to restrain her and calm her down but it really was too much for me in my state and by that time John had disappeared into the bedroom taking with him my bottle of vodka.

Fortunately, soon afterwards, a gentleman arrived at the door. Dawn was about to embark on a tour throughout the country and he was concerned with arranging suitable venues for her. He too was a spiritualist.

I explained that I was merely an acquaintance who came to Dawn for healing, after which he too did his best to try and comfort her.

"I'm not going to give up my religion," she sobbed to him.

"No, because you know it's there. Your daughter is with you now," he replied.

"She's not with me now," Dawn cried out.

"You know very well that she was out of her body immediately it happened," he said, "and now she's in a spiritual hospital where souls go when they have passed violently and need a rest." Little John, having just woken up, then came rushing into the room. He clung to his sobbing mother and Dawn said, "I love my son."

We both suggested that a doctor should come and sedate her, but she adamantly refused. However, the gentleman gave her a sedative which, for some reason or other, he carried around with him, and she was soon fast asleep with little John still clinging to her.

As soon as everything was peaceful we both sat down and chatted.

"Are you a spiritualist?" he asked.

"No," I replied, "I'm a Christian and I'm not interested in trying to contact the dead. But I believe in an afterlife in a different dimension with a spiritual body where we continue to progress. St Paul says we have a spiritual and celestial body."

He nodded and said, "Then you believe in spiritual healing?"

"Oh yes," I replied emphatically. "I believe that all inspiration whether it is music, art, poetry or whatever, comes from above and I certainly believe in spiritual healing. Christ says with God all things are possible."

At that point there was a knock on the door of the flat. The gentleman opened the door and a young lady was ushered in. For the last couple of months she had attended Dawn's development class and she had got to know both John and Dawn very well—certainly more than either of us did and when she saw the state they were both in she revealed the fact that they were both alcoholics. "Why do you think they both go to Alcoholics Anonymous and take drugs to help them to stop drinking? The only time Dawn doesn't drink is before her private readings and before her shows." And she went on, "Dawn has had a much harder life than any of us. She was brought up in a poor house in Edinburgh…sharing a dormitory with many other people, later living in the East End of London. She was the victim of a gang rape, being raped by six men and, having received no counselling, she began to drink, becoming an alcoholic some time later. She has tried to commit suicide and very nearly succeeded. That's why little John was taken away from her and made a ward of court. They told her that if she fell again they would take him away from her for good because she was an unfit mother."

We both listened in stunned silence at what she had to say. It was indeed the most appalling catalogue of tragedies and I felt very sorry for Dawn. That was the reason, of course, why she had so adamantly refused to let us call a doctor. However, the young lady said that she would take care of little John until the situation improved. John, himself, was of course fast asleep on the bed after drinking half the bottle of vodka. The gentleman left the flat soon afterwards and I told the young lady I would visit the flat the next day. I did so only to find that Dawn had spent the night at a friend's house and John was still drinking.

Fortunately my husband was with me, because I became aware immediately that in drink John's personality had dramatically altered. He was now very aggressive. He telephoned Dawn's friend and insisted that Dawn be brought back to the flat and we sat there talking to him until she arrived shortly afterwards. Alas, she was still parasitically drunk and obviously on a binge. There was nothing we could do so we left the flat soon afterwards.

"Good-bye Ruth," she said as we left, and that was the last time I saw her.

She did telephone me on two occasions. The first time was about 11 o'clock one night a few weeks later. "Ruth," she said, "I've done a lot for you. Would you do one little thing for me? Could you bring me some drink…anything? I'm shaking all over and I want to get some sleep."

"Where's John?" I asked.

"Oh, I've locked him out. He's a very violent man with drink," she said. "He's gone in the car taking all the drink and pills with him."

I hurriedly looked around for some whisky I might have had, but the bottle was empty and reluctantly I had to tell her that I had no drink whatsoever in the house.

"Good Bye Ruth," she said, immediately putting down the receiver. I felt I had let her down badly.

On the second occasion a few weeks later, she telephoned and said, "Ruth, I'm going on a long tour so I won't be able to give you any more healing."

I knew it wasn't the real reason, but I thanked her and John for all the kindness they had shown me.

"My daughter has recently died," she said.

"Yes, I know," I replied.

"You know?" she said in astonishment, being totally oblivious to the fact that I had come to the flat on those two days. However, I had no intention of going there again. What I had witnessed was all too much for me to cope with.

In June, I happened to glance through the local newspaper and I read that Dawn had been found dead behind a locked bedroom door with little John crying beside her. There was to be an inquest. John was said to be devastated. Some time later I read in the same newspaper that she had taken 60 tablets of the drug she had been prescribed to help her stop drinking. The verdict was suicide. She was only 31 years old.

Apparently she had predicted her own death to the newspaper reporter a week before it happened.

I telephoned John soon after reading the results of the inquest and I told him how sorry I was to hear of her untimely death. "It was too much pressure," he said, referring to her forthcoming tour.

"Who will look after little John?" I asked.

"Oh, I will…the same as I had to before," he replied.

I wished him well and sent a donation for the gravestone he wanted to erect.

Months passed. I continued to have treatment at the Liu Clinic but I hadn't been able to go for a holiday abroad that summer; I was still in too much torment. What I was experiencing in my head altered all the time, which meant that the Ch'i was going down but a considerable amount remained. I still didn't have a supply of sleeping pills at that time and I remember being in such a state one November day that I telephoned the surgery. Miss Knight answered.

"I can no longer cope," I told her simply.

"Why after a year do you suddenly find that you can't cope?" she asked.

I couldn't believe how stupid she was. Didn't she know that things are accumulative? "It's because of the Ch'i in my head," I replied as patiently as I could.

"Oh, it's the same old thing," she said in her usual bored manner. "It's all emotional stress and strain."

I just put down the receiver—it was hopeless trying to deal with them.

A few weeks before Christmas I was given the address of a medium and healer who lived in the vicinity. I telephoned her and she gave me an appointment. She turned out to be a 75 year old lady who had just lost her husband and I felt guilty at having bothered her. She, however, was very kind to me and gave me a number of healing sessions. She had recently returned from Egypt and she said, "Don't worry about age. I'm still enjoying life." But she kept saying, "All I'm getting from the spirits with you is 'three weeks'," which she couldn't understand. But she did tell me that once my problem had gone it would never return and she showed great sympathy for me when I told her the extent of my suffering—the fact that I had to be put to sleep as early as 2 p.m. because I could bear it no longer. By that time, thank God, I had managed to obtain a supply of sleeping tablets. If I hadn't had those to rely on I really don't know what would have happened. She said, "You're the most difficult case I have ever had to deal with."

As for the three weeks that she kept mentioning it was probably the fact that I only went to see her until Christmastime, which was three weeks in all. She was in the process of selling her large house and I didn't want to trouble her further.

Christmas came and went—not very happily for me. It was the second Christmas I had spent with the wretched Ch'i still in my head. I had been attending Dr Liu's clinic for almost a year and had all the treatment possible cupping, moxibustion, massage and herbs—but although he was always helpful, attending the clinic two or three times a week had become a strain. We had to travel through heavy traffic to get there and back. It was a nightmare.

I had tried to contact Giovanni sometime before Christmas but was told that he was in China studying herbal medicine. Now, however, I wanted desperately to find an acupuncturist who lived in the vicinity so that I could drive myself there without bothering my husband. I looked through the Yellow Pages and found the name of an acupuncturist who lived locally. I told him what the problem was and he adamantly refused to treat me.

"There are so many points I wouldn't dream of treating you," he said. But when I mentioned that I had initially received treatment from Giovanni he said enthusiastically, "He was my tutor."

"Then why don't you contact him and ask him what treatment he gave me? He was in China, but he may have returned by now," I said.

He agreed to do that, and when I telephoned him again a few days later he said that he had spoken to Giovanni and was now prepared to treat me.

He was a part-time acupuncturist, having another part-time occupation. He had only recently become qualified to treat acupuncture and he certainly wasn't skilled like Dr Liu or Giovanni, but I was prepared to give it a try. Alas, after a few treatments he had altered the way the Ch'i behaved in my head—it now gave me no peace, and furthermore I began to feel a force that rose from my feet and up into my head similar to the gale force wind I had initially experienced. On one occasion I went to bed and my heart started beating so rapidly I couldn't breathe and the force rushed up from my feet. I managed to get out of bed but I was rolling on the floor curled up like a ball and gasping for breath. I don't know why I was reacting to his treatment so badly, but later I was told that to change treatments was fatal, which proved to be the case and I was forced to stop going to the acupuncturist.

Because I was now getting very little peace, my emotional state was beginning to deteriorate rapidly. But again it was, thank God, for the sleeping pills, which got me through it at that time.

I telephoned Tina, the lady who had initially also given me acupuncture, but when I told her I still had Ch'i in my head she replied curtly, "Oh, you think too much about the Ch'i. Go for a holiday and it will go!"

She, it seemed, had lost all interest and patience with me. But she was proved wrong. Alas, it wasn't that simple.

In desperation I telephoned Giovanni and he agreed to see me. My husband carne with me. I told him what had happened and he said, "You've had too much acupuncture and you shouldn't change treatments." He agreed to give me treatment that day because I told him about the force I was experiencing, but he refused to give me any more saying, "You should try another method of healing." He gave me the name of a man who specialised in homeopathy. But before leaving he said to my husband, "I don't know why the Ch'i is taking so long to go." However, when my husband telephoned him again soon afterwards, he was told, very abruptly, that I should be taken to see a psychiatrist! Perhaps both he and Tina no longer believed that I really did have Ch'i in the head!

I went back to Dr Liu's clinic for a few treatments, but when I told him what had happened he too warned me of the dangers of changing treatments. I decided to have a rest from acupuncture altogether and see what happened. The fact was, I just couldn't face any more needles being stuck into me. I had begun to cry bitterly at every treatment.

Being entirely on my own again I decided to look around for a healer and I found a lady called Sandy who advertised in the Psychic News. I telephoned her and found that she lived only a short distance from me. She turned out to be a genuinely kind and decent person.

I began visiting her in her home where she would comfort me and give me healing and, being also a medium, she would tell me what she had picked up. On my first visit she said, "My guide said that it will go." On a subsequent visit she said, "I can see an aeroplane. You are going abroad this year." Later she told me, "There's a reason for all your suffering. You will be able to help people in the future."

I'm afraid at that time I couldn't foresee the possibility of that happening, but we never know what's around the comer. God's ways are not our ways. She very kindly lent me a book called *Sai Messages for You and Me*, Volume 1, which was written by Lucas Ralli who, some time later, I was privileged to meet. Sai Barber is a Hindu mystic—a man of spiritual enlightenment and deep compassion. His miracles are mostly healing but he also apports objects, i.e. materialisation and dematerialisation of objects, some of which I was also privileged to see. With a twist of his hand he is able to bring rings, jewels or whatever out of the air and a sacred ash called vibhuti drops from his palms in bucketfuls. Sandy had managed to obtain some ash and she dipped her finger into the plastic container and rubbed it across my forehead.

Because of my deteriorating emotional state, I began telephoning clairvoyants who advertised in Prediction. And, as with my telephoning acupuncturists at random, it proved to be an unwise thing to do. One lady I telephoned advertised as a colour therapist and mystic. She agreed to see me right away which was on a Friday.

I drove to her house and she took me to an upstairs room which was her healing sanctuary. Drawings of her guides were pinned to the wall along with a 'picture' of Christ. She seemed very sympathetic when I told her how much I was suffering, which was obvious to everyone. You only had to look at my face.

She told me to sit facing the 'picture' of Christ whilst she said a prayer, after which she proceeded to give me colour healing.

She told me how to shut down my chakra centres by simply thinking of them each in turn and locking the door with a key. "It's as simple as that," she said. "I was in hospital very ill, depleted and exhausted before I was told how to shut down. Now I'm all right." And she went on, "I have made the blind see and the deaf hear. Come again on Monday and I'll see you then. Meanwhile take this pentagrarn; it will ward off evil spirits." It was a tiny pentagram on a chain.

"How much do I owe you?" I enquired.

"Healing is free," she said.

Monday came and I went to see her again.

"What can I do for you?" she asked irritably. Her whole attitude had changed towards me, for now she was cold and quite nasty and she demanded back the pentagram she had lent me. I quickly gave it back to her and without thinking I blurted out, "Would you give me a reading?"

"Very well," she said sharply, and began laying cards on the table. She then spent a whole hour talking what seemed total mumbo jumbo to me. There was nothing that made sense. Towards the end her voice became hoarse and she said, "It always does this. The spirits use my voice box." She gathered together her cards and snapped, 'That's forty five pounds."

I was completely taken aback. I had never paid that for a reading before, even with the top psychics, and I said, "That's a lot of money."

"I could have charged you fifty pounds with healing," she replied sharply.

Healing was supposed to have been free, but I didn't bother to argue with her. I just quickly wrote out a cheque and left. I felt she had taken advantage of an obviously emotionally distraught person. But that wasn't the only bad experience I had at the time. There was another clairvoyant who advertised in Prediction and her advert began: "I am blessed by God with the gift of prophecy to help others..." and so on.

She gave telephone readings, but when I telephoned her she seemed more concerned about giving me her address where I could send my "donation" and she kept repeating, "You've had so many minutes. You've had so many minutes." However, she told me to phone the following morning at 10 a.m. and she would have an astrological chart ready for me. I did telephone a number of times but the line was always engaged, so I didn't bother again until a few weeks later when I telephoned her again hoping we could just carry on where we left off. But immediately she realised who I was she screamed, "You didn't pay me. Get off the line! I can't link up with you." She was almost hysterical and she slammed down the receiver. So much for her being blessed by God to help others!

I told Sandy of my experiences and she was appalled by their behaviour. These people are more of a menace than anything else. They must know that the majority of people who consult them are emotionally distraught for some reason or another and need to be treated with the utmost care, not blasted away. Anyhow, once again I had to learn my lesson the hard way and from then on I decided to contact clairvoyants who had a good reputation, and my opportunity came soon afterwards.

CHAPTER 13

It was late January and I happened to be passing a bookshop that had 'Closing down sale' on the windows. I went in and browsed around the bookshelves. A book entitled The Spirit Calls caught my eye. It was the autobiography of Peter Lee, the well-known clairvoyant. I bought it and read it as soon as I arrived home. I was very impressed; he was without doubt a highly gifted psychic. I didn't know where to contact him so I telephoned the publishers and they gave me his telephone number. I rang the number and his assistant answered. He gave me an early appointment because I had stressed the urgency of it. He probably didn't need to be told, having sensed the desperation in my voice.

The appointment was for 4 p.m. on a Monday in January 1988. We drove to the flat and, arriving early, went for a cup of coffee at a coffee shop close by. I remember being in a terrible state sitting there. My whole body shook from the acupuncture and the Ch'i raged in my head, but I was determined to keep the appointment.

After arriving back at the house his assistant led me up a flight of stairs to Peter Lee's apartment. He was still with another client so I sat in the waiting area and bought a tape from his assistant, having forgotten to bring my own. Soon, Peter Lee came out of his room and when he had bade farewell to his client he came over to me and greeted me cordially. He led me into a fairly large room and seated me comfortably in an armchair close to a roaring fire. He took my tape and put it into his cassette recorder. Then, holding a microphone in his hand he sat down and began to speak. He said, "When I give a reading, unless I am asked to concentrate on anything specific I give things as they come to me. If there's anything you can't understand, or don't relate to and you wish me to go further and deeper, please stop me straight away and not ten minutes later, otherwise I won't know what I'm talking about. On the other hand, if there are things you do understand then please say so." He went on to say, "I say 'I' when I mean 'you' because I work quickly from vibrations. I dodge around the time sequence. I will invite questions at the end and it does help to hear your voice occasionally."

When the preliminaries were over, I sat there praying that he would have good news for me. He was reputedly very accurate. He began, "You've been through a lot of strain and confusion. Have you been back and forth for treatment?"

"Yes," I replied, becoming immediately very emotional. "I want to know when will it all end?"

"Did they apply heat somewhere? Why can I feel heat?" he asked.

"I've been having acupuncture," I told him and he nodded. It fitted.

"Do you suffer from migraine?" he questioned, "I can feel a heaviness in the head."

"No," I said and I went on to tell him everything that had happened to me. I told him how the Ch'i had been pushed into my head by the Taiwan acupuncturist and that for over a year acupuncturists had been trying to channel the energy down to various other parts of the body.

"I've been in terrible torment since it happened," I told him, beginning to sob quietly.

He looked concerned but carried on with his reading. "Yes, it's like total agitation all the time—everything grinds, there is no harmony," he said. "They are trying to suck it down again aren't they? But it is going. They are channelling it out, but there's still a lot there. Let me see now, I'm afraid it's not around the corner but it's soon.... we are talking about this year. After June, it seems to be clearing. It seems as if something has washed through the head." Then he added, "It will go."

"Will it go?" I pleaded.

"Oh, I can promise you that it will go. It's going at the moment," he assured me.

"Shall I keep on with the acupuncture?" I asked.

"Oh, I'm afraid you might have to. They have to undo what they have done wrong, but the main thing is once it goes it will never come back."

"I don't think I can last until June, it's six month's time. I may be forced to take my life," I said through my sobs.

"You'll only have to come back and go through it again," he replied. "But you won't give in I can promise you that. This is your last year of suffering, that's for sure."

After the assurances that the Ch'i would eventually go he began telling me other things. "I can see you going on a long journey. It's across the Atlantic. Not this year, but the following year or the beginning of the year after," he said

"I've been to America twice," I told him.

"You liked it," he said, "and you'll like it again. But at the moment you have no enthusiasm for anything. But you will, you'll see."

"Am I going abroad this year?" I asked dubiously.

"You will go abroad this year, but I don't feel it will be very far. I feel you will go to the warm Atlantic—where the Mediterranean meets the Atlantic, possibly Portugal or Spain." He paused and then added, "In spite of all this suffering you will have a long life. It will teach you a lot because somehow you will assist in the alleviation of suffering of others."

Sandy had said the same thing, but again I couldn't see how that could possibly come about. He went on, "I also feel that the contrast for you when it is over will be greatly appreciated and you will live more. I'm afraid you have to suffer it alone, but as I have stressed, you won't give in. Let them undo what they have done."

"Can you see a book?" I asked.

"I can see material passed on, which is probably a book," he replied. "It will tell of your suffering, and your victory, but that is to come. I also feel that you will be a person who people will want to speak to because there are individuals being told continually that there is nothing wrong with them and they too are suffering greatly. They will only be too pleased to have someone pioneer the way. Doctors, if they couldn't

explain anything decided it wasn't there...but it was a physical thing."
How right he was.

The reading ended after about half an hour and I paid his fee and left
clasping my treasured tape. I would play it over and over again when I
felt in need of reassurance.

I tried at that time to contact Edward Fricker, the healer

who had told me "You're going to be fine" but by that time I learned
that he had sadly passed away. I am sure that he, as a person, and his
great gift of healing will be greatly missed. He ;was a lovely human being.

Soon afterwards I wrote a letter to Ray and Joan Branch who run the
Harry Edwards Healing Sanctuary in Surrey. I told them of all my troubles and a week later I received a letter from them. They said that they
would put me on their absent healing list, which I was grateful for, and
gave me the names and telephone numbers of two healers who lived in
South London. I contacted one healer, a gentleman, but he lived too far
away. I couldn't possibly manage to see him. However, I then contacted
the other healer. She turned out to be a 93 year old lady a Miss Ethel
Bailey and she only lived a short distance away from me.

"We hold healing sessions on Fridays," she said, "but you can come
this afternoon if it's urgent."

I felt that it was urgent and made an appointment to see her at 3 p.m.
that afternoon.

My husband drove me the short distance to her tiny flat on the
ground floor of a block of flats. She was a dear, sweet old lady, still
mobile and living on her own. Regarding her family she said, "I don't
see them. They just don't want to know," which seemed incredible; she
was such a lovely person.

When we were comfortably seated she went off into the kitchen to
make us both a cup of tea. She soon came back with a tray full of cups
and saucers and a teapot. I thought she might trip, but she managed it
very well and laid it on a small table.

She seated herself and began pouring the tea, telling us at the same time of her life as a healer. Her mind was remarkably lucid.

"I worked with Tom Johannson at the SAGB for ten years," she told us. 'Now he travels all over the world. I wish I could go with him, but at my age…" She went on, "You know I've seen grown men cry when I've healed them."

As soon as we had finished our tea, she took us into an adjoining room, which she had turned into a sanctuary. On the walls were pictures of her spirit doctors and there was a tiny altar on which were lighted candles.

It was so peaceful and we all said a little prayer.

"Look," she said afterwards, "this is what Sai Barber apported for me. I was looking on my table, sorting things out, when I saw this," she pointed to a ring on her little finger, "it's silver with a purple colour and it's very pure. It has the leaf imprinted on it. I found that it fitted my little finger." Her face lit up with delight as she said it.

Afterwards, she led us back into the sitting room and began looking through her diaries. "I'm going to give you the name and telephone number of Lucas Ralli. Get in touch with him. We worked together at the SAGB for years. He used to have a healing sanctuary in his home but he doesn't any longer.

Lucas Ralli was the author of *Sai Messages for You and Me* and I couldn't believe she was telling me to contact him.

"He's a real gentleman, his father was a 'Sir' you know," she said proudly.

We bade farewell to the old lady, promising to come on Friday evening for healing, but it turned out that I was in too much distress to go and sadly I had to cancel the appointment. However, after leaving Miss Bailey's flat I telephoned Lucas Ralli and told him that Miss Bailey had kindly given me his name and telephone number and asked if it was possible for me to have an appointment with him.

"I no longer have a sanctuary," he said. "I leave that to younger people. I am very busy, I work from 4.30 every morning until 8 at night, but I'll give you a ring tomorrow and see when I can fit you in."

I thanked him. He was clearly doing Miss Bailey a favour.

As promised he did ring the following day. "Come and see me tomorrow at 1 a.m. and I'll give you an hour," he said.

It was a Saturday and my husband and I made our way to his house in town. We had been warned that there was no parking space anywhere near the house so, whilst David went off to find somewhere to park I walked up to the large house and rang the bell.

"Who is it?" I heard a lady's voice say over the entry phone.

"It's Mrs Barrett," I answered, and I was required to repeat it a few times. A lady in a nightdress soon opened the door.

"I was in bed, I've got gastric flu. I'm sorry I took so long in coming, but my name was Mrs Barrett before I married again and I got confused. Let's go downstairs," she said.

She led me downstairs to the sitting room and opened the wooden shutters.

"Lucas is having a bath, but he won't be long," she said. "Sit down and make yourself comfortable." I sat on the settee.

It wasn't long before Lucas Ralli came into the sitting room. He was a rather lean, middle-aged man, very distinguished looking and, as Miss Bailey had said, he was a real gentleman. I appreciated the fact that he had given up his precious time to see me.

He sat in an armchair and began asking many questions as to the nature of my distress. I couldn't call it an illness. I told him everything I could. But, like everybody else, I think he was a bit sceptical when I told him I had too much Ch'i in the head. "It's not the easiest of cases," he said, "but I wouldn't embark on another year of acupuncture if I were you." He was probably thinking that it had failed to get rid of what was in my head.

My husband then arrived and he too was made comfortable in an armchair. Lucas Ralli exchanged a few words with him and then it was time for the healing session. He asked me to sit on an upright chair and relax as best I could. Unfortunately it wasn't one of my better days and I was in some distress, but I tried not to show it.

He stood behind me and placed his hands on my head. "I only heal once," he said. "Some people fall asleep while I heal them but they are mostly men, but you may feel drowsy." He closed his eyes and breathed deeply, moving his hands to my shoulders.

The healing session lasted half an hour. I didn't go to sleep or even feel drowsy. The Ch'i sizzling away as it was probably prevented me from fully relaxing.

I sat facing a wall on which was a large picture of a man who I knew to be Sai Barber and when the healing session had finished and I was once again seated on the settee, I mentioned that I had read the book "Sai messages for you and me", Volume 1, written of course by himself, and had seen ash which had reputedly dropped from the palms of Sai Barber's hands.

"Are you interested in Sai Barber?" he said, enthusiastically. I nodded. "I'll get you some ash," he said, immediately getting up from his seat and going out of the room. He returned with the ash, which was in a small plastic container.

Handing it to me he said, "I would put some on your tongue in the morning and at night."

I told him I would do that and then asked, "Did it drop from his hands?"

"Not that particular ash," he replied, "but it has been blessed."

"Miss Bailey showed me the ring that Sai Barber apported for her," I told him.

"I've got two," he replied, pointing to a silver ring on his finger. "I can't wear the other ring because it's broken. I also have a leaf which was apported. It has a 'picture' of Jesus on it holding a lamb. I went out of my office one day and when I came back I found it lying on my desk. I'll show it to you when we go upstairs." And he added, "I've seen Sai Barber in India on five occasions."

Referring to his book "Sai messages for you and me" I asked, "How do you receive the messages? Does he dictate them to you?"

"Oh no," he replied, "Sai Barber once said that he was like a radio channel and anyone could tune in, so I thought I would give it a try. I just sit down quietly and the thoughts come into my head and I write them down. I would never be able to write such beautiful words myself," He smiled at me and then went on, "I typed the book out with two fingers. It's sold at cost price—I don't want any royalties. The first book sold 3,000 copies and the second one, Volume II, has so far sold 1,000 copies. It is going to be translated and sold abroad. You know, years ago, a medium told me that I would write a book that would be sold all over the world." He paused and then continued, "I could have written a book on healing but I didn't. I used to heal with Tom Johannson at the SAGB. I did it for years. He's the real king pin, but some people can go from healer to healer and still not be healed. I don't do any healing now—I haven't got the time. I'm the representative of Sai Barber in this country and now for the whole of Europe. That takes a lot of work. I'm up at 4.30 am. and I work all day."

"Have you seen Sai Barber perform any miracles?" I asked.

"Yes," he replied, "I've seen him apport a beautiful diamond ring for a lady and once there was a girl of about eight or ten standing close by him and he turned his hand, the way he does, and a kind of fudge dropped on the floor. We all picked it up and ate it. It was delicious."

"Has he healed anybody?" I asked.

"Well there was one man who was paralysed from the neck down. Sai Barber said to him, "I can heal you but you are paying back Karma and you'll only have to come back and do it again. The man chose not to be healed and seemed so happy."

"Is he ever going to come to Europe?" I asked.

"Oh no," he replied hastily, "I don't think we are ready for him," which was probably true. He went on to say, "You know the famous direct voice medium Leslie Flint used to live next door. He was my neighbour for many years."

As we were mounting the stairs on our way out David reminded him of his promise to show us the leaf that had been apported to him by Sai Barber.

Immediately Lucas Ralli went into his study and brought out the leaf, which was now in a wooden frame. He said, "I asked Sai Barber if the leaf was happy in the wooden frame and he replied, "Frame not important but picture is."

I held the precious frame and we both marvelled at the leaf with its 'picture' of Jesus holding a lamb painted on it.

"If you hold it up to the light it's transparent," Lucas Ralli said. But we weren't able to do that, of course, because of the frame.

He also brought out of his study the book, "Sai messages for you and me", Volume II, which he gave to me along with the picture of the leaf, which I treasure.

I was asked to contact him in three week's time and let him know howl was faring, and he added, "We will be leaving this house in a couple of months and moving to the country. It's more peaceful there."

He led us to the door and stood waving to us as we walked away from the house. He seemed a happy, contented man and I envied him. It was a wonderful way to work for God.

Alas, I didn't contact him in three week's time as he had suggested. I felt I couldn't disappoint him by telling him that I was not significantly any better. The Ch'i remained in my head and my emotional state was now at its lowest point.

CHAPTER 14

In early March, because I was so emotionally distraught I went again to the surgery and saw Miss Stevens. She gave me a letter to take to Maudsley Hospital Emergency Clinic, but for some reason or other I didn't go. She had, however, given me a week's supply of chlorapromazine tablets. At first she had said, "I will give you two tablets a day and you'll have to go to the chemist each day to pick them up."

It was so stupid and unnecessary that I protested vehemently and she eventually said, "Very well I'll give you a week's supply, but no more."

In my anxiety I began to search for yet another acupuncturist, so I telephoned the British Institute of Acupuncture. I spoke to a Chinese gentleman and I told him that I had too much Ch'i in my head as a result of having acupuncture for tinnitus. He seemed genuinely concerned and told me to come to the Institute the following morning at 9.30 a.m.

The Institute was close to Victoria Station and we travelled there by train, which was very convenient for us. Alas, right from the beginning he infuriated me. He insisted on knowing the name of the acupuncturist who had treated me for tinnitus and when I told him he said, "I know him socially. Did you tell him that things were getting worse?"

"Of course," I replied. He didn't answer; so I went on to tell him that I had received treatment from Dr Liu for a year. "He's been channeling the Ch'i out of my head."

"I'm a better acupuncturist than either of those two," he said smugly, "I've had twenty years' experience."

Dr Liu wouldn't like that I thought to myself. After all he has had thirty years' experience and he is a medical doctor. However, I went on to tell him that initially I had received treatment from Giovanni but now he was refusing to give me any more treatment.

"Why did you leave him?" he asked in surprise. He obviously respected Giovanni.

"I couldn't have regular treatment with him because he was always so booked up. That's why I went to Dr Liu," I replied.

Immediately he retorted, "Well, if you left him and went to Dr Liu for a year I am not surprised he refused to have anything more to do with you."

I thought it was a childishly petty attitude to take and furthermore it was not correct. Giovanni had not refused to treat me because I had been to Dr Lin's clinic but because he felt I had had enough acupuncture, which was probably true. I am certain he would not have been that small minded.

"Now," he said, "I don't want to hear any more about Ch'i." I sighed. What was I going to say if I wasn't allowed to mention Ch'i? After all, that's what it was!

"Give me a year," he said, "and I'll make you better." I shuddered at the thought of another year of acupuncture. It was totally unrealistic.

"Undress to your panties and lie on the bed face downward," he said, and then left the room whilst I undressed.

I lay waiting for him on the bed, wondering where it was all going to end. I was beginning to lose all hope.

He came into the room and placed needles at the base of my skull and on my legs. I asked him what treatment he was giving me. Dr Lin and Giovanni had always tried to explain to me what they were attempting to do, but he didn't answer, which further irritated me. He simply ignored my question.

When he had finished needling me, however, he walked out of the room, leaving me pondering over my cruel fate. Twenty minutes later he returned and took out the needles. He said, "I want to see you once every week," and without further ado he walked out of the room again.

I quickly dressed and went upstairs to where my husband was waiting. I made an appointment for the following week and paid his fee.

The next week at the appointed time I went again to the clinic and received treatment from the gentleman. But after the initial interview he spoke only to my husband. If I attempted to speak or ask a question he didn't answer and just looked through me as if I didn't exist.

Naturally, that kind of behaviour and attitude to me was intolerable. Even though I clearly was in the most deplorable emotional state I always had my senses, my mind was not affected in any way and I wanted to be treated as the intelligent woman that I am. Unfortunately, because of his behaviour towards me, I showed my frustration and irritation, which did nothing to help matters. Nevertheless, I made an appointment for the following week, but because of the state I was in I cancelled it. I felt if I saw him again and he refused to speak to me I was likely to scream the place down.

Tai Ch'i I knew to be excellent. Dr Liu of course held classes on it at his clinic and Giovanni had recommended it. It consists of slow movements, which apparently balances mind and body. The classes at Dr Liu's clinic were at an inconvenient time for me. They were held in the evening. I thought the movements might help my predicament so I telephoned a Chinese gentleman who was a Tai Ch'i expert. I told him that I had Ch'i in the head and wondered if there were any exercises I could do that would help my condition. To my astonishment he agreed to come to the house, travelling all the way from North London. I was thrilled.

He turned out to be a short, stocky-looking gentleman. He came into the house and sat himself down on the settee and immediately said, "Now I will see what's really wrong with you." He went on, "You can't possibly feel Ch'i in the head. We've got Ch'i in every part of the body. Look!" He rubbed his hands together, "That's Ch'i, but you can't see or feel it."

And he went on from there to further sneer at me until I had had enough and told him to leave. He had travelled all that way just to ridicule the fact that I told him I had Ch'i in the head. To him it had to be something else, probably my mind. But he was wrong. It had to be

Ch'i in my head—it couldn't be anything else and the manner in which it finally left proved it.

Because I wasn't getting any relief from the torment I was becoming more and more distraught. I used to pace the house sobbing all day. As I have stated, lying down or even sitting down made everything worse. Pressure on the spine had a distinct effect on the Ch'i. I went again to see Miss Stevens and I asked for another letter to attend Maudsley Emergency Clinic—a letter that was more accurate—I knew that in her last letter she had written that I had a psychosis and needed major tranquilizers pins God knows what treatment and that I had threatened to commit suicide several times, none of which was correct and I told her so. She then set about writing a letter in which she stated that I complained of having Ch'i or energy in the head which was indeed a dramatic turn about for her.

I wasn't able to go that day because the nursing staff were staging a one-day strike, but I went first thing the following day.

I saw a young lady psychiatrist who took down the usual details and seemed to understand perfectly well that I really was in physical torment. She seemed very concerned about what might happen to me. "I've given you a prescription for a major tranquilizer. You are to take a large dosage for the time being and you are to get more from your GP when they run out."

"She won't give them to me," I cried out, and I told her what Miss Stevens had said about me having to go to the chemist each day to pick up two tablets.

"She'll give them to you," she replied sharply.

I took the tablets as prescribed but, alas, they affected my vision. Everything was blurred and I couldn't function at all so I stopped taking them and was once again back to square one. My husband was so concerned that he telephoned the GP. It was Sunday, so he had to telephone the emergency number. Miss Stevens answered and when told of my distress she came immediately to the house. In fairness to her, she always responded to an emergency by coming to the house.

She quickly wrote out a letter for me to take to St Thomas' Hospital Emergency Clinic and we drove there immediately. I was required to wait what seemed like an eternity before being seen by the psychiatrist. My torment was so great that I was obliged to pace up and down the corridor, almost collapsing. When the doctor did arrive I was asked to go into a small cubicle where he asked the usual long list of questions which I could barely answer. He was a very young man but he could see that it was indeed an emergency and that I was desperately in need of some sort of help if I was to survive the terrible ordeal I was condemned to live through.

He suggested I went to a psychiatric hospital not far away and stay the night so that I could be observed and given treatment.

I agreed and so he telephoned the hospital to see if they had a bed— they did and so he quickly wrote a letter for me to give them. We drove there straight away. On arrival at the hospital the lady psychiatrist took me into a small room and, after asking a long list of questions said, "I suggest you stay the night." I tentatively agreed to do so but I didn't know how I was going to cope—especially having to get through the night without the aid of a sleeping pill. I wasn't sure that they would give me a sedative.

The nurse in charge had told my husband that it was better if he left the hospital, which he did. She then led me into a small communal sitting room and left me sitting there alone. I began to sob and sob almost hysterically. Eventually the nurse carne back and said, "You must stay the night so that we can treat you. You're a young woman and you've got a lot to live for." But I kept on sobbing.

I began pacing the corridors for some considerable time and then I went into the sleeping area and tried lying on the bed but, as usual, the Ch'i in my head was worse and I sobbed even louder. A rather disturbed lady came into the room and started shouting at me, "Shut up, shut up," she kept repeating. It was hopeless.

I begged the lady psychiatrist to give me a sleeping pill, but she adamantly refused. "You can't have one until ten o'clock tonight. We have to observe normal sleeping hours," she insisted. That was the end for me. I immediately rang my husband and asked him to take me home.

He soon arrived at the hospital and it was a considerable relief to me to know that I was going home. The lady psychiatrist, however, seemed to understand the situation and she said to me before I left, "Do what you usually do to get through the night." I just nodded.

The following morning I went again to the hospital and asked to see the lady psychiatrist. They agreed and I was asked to go to the Out-Patients Department. I waited there some time before being seen by her and also the consultant psychiatrist. She had discussed my case with him beforehand.

"We have come to the conclusion that you don't need to be an in-patient," the consultant said, "but we are giving you chlorapromazine tablets to take. You must take them. I think you should also attend the Day Centre one or two days a week."

I declined that suggestion. How could I possibly attend a Day Centre in my condition. Like everyone else they failed to comprehend that I was truly in physical torment. If I had been in pain I would no doubt be given painkillers or even morphine, but I had no relief from my tor-ment—it was with me all day and every day. The only relief I had was when I was asleep and then I had to wake up to face the same problem. It was truly hell.

Not long afterwards, my husband once again called the GP. It was on a Sunday and he probably thought that what he was doing was for the best. Miss Stevens answered the telephone and she said she would come imme-diately to the house. I was in bed at the time and she sat on the bed and said matter-of-factly, "You've got three choices; either you go to the local psychiatric clinic, or to the hospital, or I will impose Section 4."

I had never heard of Section 4, so to satisfy her I said I would go to the local clinic. I thought that she had no right to tell me that I had three choices. How dare she order me to choose one of them. I, after all, hadn't even telephoned her. I had been asleep in bed. As soon as she left, however, I bathed, dressed and my husband drove me to the clinic, which was very close to home.

The psychiatrist turned out to be an Indian lady. She once again asked me many questions and I answered them all correctly.

"Do you want an injection to calm you down?" she asked.

"Why not?" I murmured, and nodded my head. She then proceeded to give me an injection that hurt so much I groaned loudly. My arm seemed to be on fire. She then left the room to have a word with my husband.

"Do you think she should be admitted to a psychiatric hospital," she had asked him. He unwittingly had answered simply, "Yes." Sitting quietly in my chair I was unaware of what had taken place and was astounded to see a woman and a burly young man almost immediately rush into the room, locking the doors behind them. Immediately I panicked and began to struggle in a vain attempt to open the doors. When I found I couldn't open them I began to hit out at the woman, but the burly man held my arms. I kept on struggling, falling to the floor, grazing my knees and ripping my stockings. My husband was nowhere to be seen and he was totally unaware of what was taking place. Since there was no point in struggling any further I submitted. Soon afterwards two ambulance men came into the room and one of them said with a smug smile, "If you don't come quietly with us we will send for the police." I could have killed him. It was an incredible situation. There I was being forced, against my will, into a psychiatric hospital, when it was the last place I felt I should be. I needed help but being locked in a psychiatric hospital was not the answer. I still feel angry at what happened. The wretched Indian doctor had got it all wrong. She had imposed Section 4.

"You'd better come along too," said one of the ambulance men to the man and woman. He was obviously expecting trouble. I was thereupon taken to the ambulance and bundled in. I felt like a criminal. We then drove off at speed to a South London psychiatric hospital. I could see my husband following in the car. I was no danger to myself or anyone else, so how was it possible that I could be forcibly taken, against my will, to a psychiatric hospital? But there I was, sitting in the ambulance between two hefty men who were making sure I didn't escape. It was ridiculous and unnecessary.

The ambulance soon arrived at the hospital and we all alighted. I was then escorted to a door on the ground floor that had to be opened with a large key. It was terrifying. I was taken through the door and into a large room and I stood looking at the scene before me.

The room or ward was dismal and bare with very disturbed patients wandering around, shouting out. It was how I imagined hell to be.

My husband then arrived and he too was considerably shaken at what had happened. But he was now powerless to help me.

"They won't keep you long," said the woman as she walked out of the ward leaving me standing there. But the thought of even spending one night in the place made me shudder and I began to shake uncontrollably. Fortunately a young doctor immediately appeared on the scene.

"I'll take you upstairs," he said, and we immediately left the ward. The heavy door was locked behind us. It was a relief to get out of the place. In comparison the ward upstairs was quite cheery. The communal sitting room had armchairs and a television set. Some of the patients looked withdrawn but seemed harmless enough.

I was taken to a small room that adjoined the dining area while my husband waited outside. The young psychiatrist asked the usual long list of questions which I was beginning to know off by heart and at the end he concluded, "There's nothing wrong with your mind," which was something I could have told him straight away. "However," he went on' "it is my opinion that you have tinnitus in the head and that's permanent." I felt it was an insensitive remark to make and furthermore not correct. However, I didn't bother to argue with him. I was now resigned to the fact that it was very difficult for some doctors to accept the fact that Ch'i existed at all, let alone the fact that I had too much in my head.

"You've been brought here under Section 4 and we can keep you here for three nights, but if you promise not to leave the hospital I'll put you upstairs where there is no lock on the door," he said.

Without hesitating I replied, "I promise not to leave the hospital." Anything was better than having to stay downstairs with those poor demented souls and I was grateful that he had at least used his common sense on that issue. He then went out of the room and spoke to my husband. "There's nothing wrong with her mind," he repeated, "but if she leaves the hospital the police will only have to bring her back!" It really was ludicrous. If I hadn't been in such torment I might well have found it amusing, but it was anything but amusing and I despaired at being forced to stay in the place for three days.

My husband then left the hospital to bring my nightdress and the necessary toiletries while I went into the communal sitting room. I did my best to relax but the Ch'i was sizzling away at the top of my head and it was impossible for me to read the newspapers or watch television, so once again I found myself pacing the corridors sobbing my heart out. One of the nurses came up to me and told me to be quiet. "We've got a lot of disturbed patients here," she said sharply.

"Well that's your problem," I retorted, "I shouldn't be here, I'm in physical torment," but she took no notice whatsoever of what I said.

My husband soon arrived with a suitcase full of the things I needed. He left immediately but promised to return in the afternoon. I managed to eat some lunch, but afterwards I began pacing the corridors once more. I asked one of the nurses if I could have a sleeping pill, but as usual she refused. "You can have one to go to bed tonight," she said. So, yet again they took no notice of the fact that I was in considerable torment and I was just left to suffer.

My husband came back to the hospital, as promised, in the afternoon and we sat in a small room and talked. I always felt better when he was around. Re left just before tea time. The women's sleeping quarters had sixteen beds and it adjoined the sitting room, whilst the men's sleeping quarters were at the other end of the ward past the sitting room and dining area. I had been told which bed was mine and after tea I undressed and tried lying down, praying that I would go to sleep, but I failed to do so. I kept getting up and walking about.

At about 7 p.m. I was given a sedative, but it didn't work, probably because I was so distraught my mind kept going over and over the trauma of the day's events. At 10 p.m. the night nurse gave me another sedative, but I still didn't sleep and I kept getting in and out of bed. By this time the lights were off and all the other patients were in bed, some snoring away.

The night nurse came up to me and said, "You're disturbing all the other patients," and promptly led me to a small room in which was a single bed.

'Try and sleep in here," I was told.

I did try, but I began to feel very cold, so I got up and went back to my own bed. I fell asleep at about 1 a.m. out of sheer exhaustion.

I was awakened at 8 a.m. by a nurse who shouted, "Get up, it's time to get up."

I bathed, dressed and ate a substantial breakfast. Fortunately, the Ch'i in my head had died down and although I was always aware of it I was able to cope much better. I spent the morning reading all the newspapers and watching television, aware of the fact that I was being observed at all times. I was careful not to put a foot wrong, not wanting to stay there a moment longer than necessary.

That morning I saw the young psychiatrist who had interviewed me on arrival at the hospital and he said that I might he able to go home that very afternoon, but a Ugandan doctor intervened. He felt that I should see a psychologist the following day. I sighed, knowing that with all his good intentions it was a waste of my time. I knew only too well what my problem was.

That afternoon my husband came and visited me and we both thought it a good idea if we went to the canteen, which was in a separate building, but when we asked the nurse for permission our request was refused. She said, "She's under close supervision and she is not allowed to leave the building."

That night they gave we 100 mg of surmontil instead of a sedative and I managed to have a much more restful night. From then on I was required to take the drug regularly every night.

The following morning the nurse told me that the doctors and the consultant would be arriving at the hospital at 2 p.m. that afternoon and they would decide then whether or not I could go home. I couldn't bear the waiting and I kept looking at the clock. I managed to eat a little lunch but after that was over I became more and more anxious. I was beginning to panic, I wanted desperately to go home and I knew if they said I had to stay another night I might well become hysterical. My husband arrived shortly before 2 p.m. and I relaxed a little, but when I saw the doctors arriving just after 2 p.m., and amongst them the consultant I had walked out on a year or two previously, I could have collapsed. I began to shake uncontrollably and my heart thumped in my chest.

"Please God not him," I gasped, "he will definitely make me stay here."

They all assembled in a room adjoining the dining room and it was about ten minutes before we were both invited into the room. "Sit down, sit down," said the consultant with a friendly smile. However, I sensed immediately that he had recognised me and the first thing he said to me after we were seated was, "Why didn't you carry on with bolvidon? You only took it one night."

"Because it made me so dizzy and I felt as if I was going mad," I answered truthfully, and he made no further comment on the issue. But his behaviour had obviously concerned him and given him a guilty conscience, and so it should have. He had behaved abominably, without any regard to the consequences of his actions.

Coffee was then brought in on a tray and handed around. It all seemed so civilized and worlds apart from what I had experienced a day or two earlier that I relaxed a little. "Things might not be so bad," I said to myself and I took a deep breath.

We all drank our coffee and I mentioned the fact that I had a ticket for Covent Garden that night—which I did have and I hoped the consultant would respond to it, and he did, "Well we wouldn't dream of keeping you from Covent Garden," he said graciously. He was certainly doing his best to behave impeccably on this occasion. Perhaps he was trying to compensate for what had happened at our last meeting, or perhaps this time there were other doctors present, which is the more likely explanation. Anyhow, he went on to say, turning to the other doctors, "Cancel the Section 4 immediately. Rescind the order."

There was no dissent among the other doctors but the young psychiatrist who had interviewed me on arrival said, "I want to say something before she leaves. I think that she has tinnitus in the head and that it is permanent. Therefore I don't think acupuncture is going to do her any good." I knew he was completely wrong, but I made no comment. I just wanted to get out of the place.

It was agreed that I should visit the clinic regularly and see the Ugandan doctor, which I was very pleased to do. It meant that I could obtain my surmontil tablets without ever going near the wretched GPs and that really was a relief. I was given a prescription for my surmontil tablets and an appointment for the clinic. I was then allowed to go home. However, before leaving, I couldn't help but say to the consultant, "I am writing a book about my experiences, and you'll be in it." He burst out laughing, thinking possibly that it was one big joke!

As we were leaving the ward, one of the male nurses came up to my husband and said, "If it happens again you won't be allowed to visit her!" If what happens again? I had been unwillingly taken there in the first place and my husband was not likely to make the same mistake again. What had happened was a disgrace.

After a few weeks of taking the tablets my emotional state did improve to the extent that my husband telephoned the Chinese acupuncturist at the British Institute of Acupuncturists and asked if I could have an appointment, but he adamantly refused, "No, definitely not," he snapped. "She upsets me every time I see her."

"But her emotional state has improved," argued my husband.

"No," he replied. "I sympathise with her condition but I refuse to treat her again."

"Well can you recommend anyone else at the institute?" asked my husband.

"Certainly not!" was his reply and he put down the receiver. He had proved, in my opinion, to be the petty, small-minded man I had always thought him to be.

CHAPTER 15

In March 1988 I read an article in the Psychic News that told of the recent successes of the British healer Allon Bacon. It stated that he had recently cured the Chief of Traffic Police in a major French city. His police work had left him with a damaged spine and neck as well as a day and night headache. Allon had apparently said, "He came to me chewing ten aspirins a day to bear the pain." It seemed that he had similarly healed an English woman of 27 he had met in the South of France where he lived during the autumn and winter. She had had a car accident in 1973 and fell from a horse several years later and had tried osteopathy and chiropractice "without much success" she had explained.

Since Allon Bacon obviously had a great gift of healing and I was still in so much torment, I set about trying to contact him. It was now spring, so he might well be back in England. I rang up Psychic News and they gave me his address and telephone number. He lived in Brighton and I wasted no time telephoning him. A very gentle, softly spoken man answered. It was Allon Bacon. I asked if I could possibly have an appointment to see him and he answered, "Write to me asking for an appointment and I will write back and give you a time."

I did so immediately. A few days later I had a reply from him. I was given an appointment for the following Wednesday at 3 p.m.

I was a bit apprehensive about the journey. I hadn't ventured so far since my terrible ordeal had begun, but it all went very smoothly. My husband drove me there and we deliberately started off early so that we could lunch in a restaurant overlooking the sea. I had been enclosed in the dark cave that Dawn had seen for so long that I had forgotten how beautiful the outside world was. I love the sea and after lunch we went for a short walk on the beach. I took long deep breaths and remembered how things used to be. I had taken everything for granted in those days, which I would probably never do again. But Peter Lee had promised that the contrast when it was over would be so greatly appreciated I would live more. I couldn't wait for that day to come.

After our stroll on the beach we set off to find the address we had been given, and without much difficulty we found the bungalow, arriving there just minutes before Allon Bacon, who had been healing at the local hospital. His face was deeply lined but he was still a handsome, imposing figure. He sported a beard. I didn't know at the time that for ten years he had been an actor, coming from a theatrical family, and began his healing when he cured himself of TB.

He led us both into his tiny bungalow that was so full of memorabilia you could hardly move around. Nevertheless, I didn't fail to notice the framed picture of the actress Vivien Leigh on the baby grand piano. Allon Bacon then asked me to sit on a stool, sitting himself on an upright chair directly behind me. My husband had managed to find a seat in an armchair by the fireplace and when we were all comfortable Allon Bacon asked in a soft, soothing voice, "What is the problem?"

I did my best to explain what had happened, but whether he believed that it was Ch'i I had in my head I don't know, for he made no comment. He gently stroked my back for about twenty minutes and then asked if I felt anything happening. I simply shook my head sadly. For all my efforts to seek healing it seemed that the Ch'i was not going to miraculously leave my head. Was I condemned to having to live with it until it finally left of its own accord? I was, and it took several more tormented years, but thank God I didn't know that at the time. Allon Bacon then asked, "What do you think about spiritual healing?"

"I think all things are possible," I replied.

"Well at least you are keeping an open mind on the subject," he said. There the session ended and we made another appointment in a week's time, but he stressed before we left, "I only heal three times and if there is no improvement I don't heal any more."

We travelled to Brighton the following week and Allon Bacon very kindly gave me healing once again, but as before nothing dramatic happened. We planned to go again but Allon Bacon, having looked through his diaries said he was heavily booked up over the Easter holidays, so we didn't make another appointment and as it turned out we never went again.

Just over a year later I read that he had been invited to Hollywood. It came about because of his successful healing of the muscular and neck problems of the direct voice medium Leslie Flint, whose guide is said to be the silent screen idol Rudolf Valentino. It seems that his friends in America wanted to know how he looked so well and Leslie Flint told them of his recent healing with Allon Bacon and they said, "Send him over!"

I was also interested to read that Vivien Leigh, whose photograph was so prominently displayed on his baby grand piano, had made her spiritual return to him days after her passing and had reappeared to him whilst he was in Hollywood. It seems he had known her during her lifetime and regarding the spiritual appearance he said, "She looked absolutely radiant."

And to Allon, who had comforted her with the assurances that she would survive bodily death, she said, "You were quite right Allon, I made a wonderful entrance. I have come to thank you."

He mentioned to me the fact that he was clairvoyant, but when I asked him to let me know what he picked up during the healing session he refused saying, "I have to concentrate all my thought and energies on healing."

A few weeks before Easter, a young gentleman called Francis had contacted me. The healer whose name I had been given by John and Ray Branch and found too inconvenient to get to had contacted him because he lived only a reasonable distance away. Francis asked to come to the house and I was only too pleased to let him come. He turned out to be a genuinely kind, compassionate gentleman and very intelligent—

everything he said was to the point and made sense. After the healing session he sat and talked to me for over an hour.

For my next healing session I arranged to go to his house when it was convenient for him, and when my husband could drive me there. We found that he was married with three lovely children; but saying something similar to Allon Bacon he said, "I will heal four times and if there is no sign of any improvement I will give you the name of a healer who is one of the best in Britain. She was my tutor."

Alas, after the fourth session nothing significant had happened so he gave me the name, address and telephone number of the lady healer. "I would go," he urged, "since it has come your way." And, after promising him that I would definitely see the lady, he asked, "Would you like to see a video film of her in action? It was a pilot film."

Enthusiastically we both said "Yes," and he immediately put the tape into the recorder. The healer looked in her sixties and we noticed that the moment she began healing her right hand would begin to shake. "It only shakes when she heals," said Francis, "it doesn't heal otherwise. She's very good with cancer. She's had it twice herself. She has an open house every Wednesday. I'll ring her and let her know you're coming."

The lady lived in Chelsea and he gave us instructions on how to find the house. I told him how grateful I was for his kindness. But before we left he returned the book "The Spirit Calls" by Peter Lee. On the occasion that he had come to the house he had noticed the book and asked to borrow it, "I read it with interest," he said. "Some of my colleagues at work have consulted him."

"What did they say about him?" I inquired eagerly.

"They said he was very accurate," he replied. It was very encouraging, since Peter Lee had stressed that the wretched Ch'i would one day leave my head. I felt so much in need of that kind of reassurance that I telephoned him once again and asked for an early appointment, even though it was Easter time.

"Come at 7 p.m. tomorrow," he said. "I can give you an appointment right away because it's holiday time."

We travelled there by car and my husband waited, as usual, outside the house. Peter Lee's assistant led me into the house and I sat quietly until he had finished with another client, but it wasn't long before I found myself seated, once again, in the armchair by the fireplace with Peter Lee sitting alongside me holding a microphone. I had brought a tape with me and he had put it into the cassette recorder. Having recognised me he quickly dispensed with the preliminaries saying, "Do you remember the explanation I gave you last time?" I just nodded. "When were you here last please?" he asked.

"In January," I replied.

"Oh it's quite recent," he said. Suddenly he paused and then went on, "Oh, it's like a phenomenal electric shock and I'm forever going..... then I get a bit of peace and then it comes back again. It's a terrible thing when you are in torment and nobody believes you. Mind you, you've had some daft doctors, but even your own family took time to realise it was all true."

"I didn't expect to live," I said.

"I will make you a promise that you will live and it will get better. But have I not told you that before?" he asked. I nodded and he continued, "Bloody acupuncture made it worse. The application that followed was worse. The doctors think that you are imagining it but it's physical. But your suffering will one day come to an end that's for sure. You see I don't play about. I can evade a question but I cannot lie. If I thought I only had something destructive to tell you I would have made an excuse not to see you. I've done it before," he stressed. And he went on' "No, it's going, I give you my word of honour that it will go and I hope that when you do get well you will protest—it's wicked. Once you are free from it all life will begin again. But it is hard for other people to know what you are going through because it's so unique to you—so special to you. I'm going to give you the name of a healer who I have just come across. He's been a healer for forty years and he's had consistent success. I'll give him a ring now." He got up immediately and rang the healer, but there was an answering machine on the healer's line so he simply gave him my telephone number and asked if he would contact me as soon as possible. He sat down again looking relieved that he had been able to do something positive to help me. I mentioned the fact that I had been given the name of another healer and intended going to see the lady, but he said, "Go to this man, he's a fantastic healer." So I promised him that I would see them both.

Once again, he told me that I would go abroad in the summer and that I would cross the Atlantic in the not too distant future, but when I looked somewhat dubious about the possibility of it all coming to pass he said, "If I see it, it will happen—otherwise I wouldn't be able to see it. I'm not a mind reader." He paused and ended the session by saying, "When it is finally over you will once again be a 100% member of the team. You have a long time on the earth plane, no way are they going to take you up there yet, you've got a lot to do. Yours is a unique kind of suffering."

He was correct; it was indeed a unique kind of suffering. The circumstances by which it had come about were unique -being on the cube whilst having acupuncture—I am convinced that that was the reason why my whole head had been filled with excess Ch'i. But what was the purpose behind it all? To me it was simply suffering for the sake of suffering since I wasn't ill in the true sense of the word and practically nobody believed that I had excess Ch'i in my head. But the fact is our bodies are made up entirely of matter and energy and energy IS the life force—without that we wouldn't be able to live.

Psychics can also see that our bodies are surrounded by vibrating energy called the aura which changes colour depending on the state of our health. So those people who dismiss energy or a force in the body as something fanciful in the mind in my opinion don't know what they are talking about. Because I mentioned Ch'i at all I was sent to the inevitable psychiatrist—to the GPs I must have had a psychosis. It has been my sad lot to actually feel this energy, the torment was very real, the suffering unique—it could only have been Ch'i!

However, around that time, apart from consulting Peter Lee, I consulted quite a few clairvoyants and mediums. I know it seems a very dangerous and unhealthy preoccupation, but such was my despair and desperation that because they gave me hope I clung to them. They could see the light at the end of the tunnel that I could only pray for. At that time it was simply a matter of keeping myself alive day by day and even worse, night by night—my torment was always a hundred times worse when I lay down—don't ask me why, perhaps someone in the world knows. But it was again thank God for the sleeping pills I had managed to obtain—not through the GPs, but I didn't have an unlimited supply so I used them sparingly. I only took them when I could bear it no longer and thought I might go mad. Unfortunately that was sometimes as early in the day as 2 o'clock in the afternoon. Looking back, I don't know how I got through it all. I know I couldn't go through the horror again.

One of the clairvoyants I saw at that time was a gentleman who called himself a Welsh African Seer. He lived in Brixton and we travelled by car for our appointment with him. We were both invited into his house and my husband was asked to make himself comfortable in the sitting room while I was led downstairs to a small room where we sat facing one another in armchairs.

When I had telephoned him for an appointment he had said, "I have a good reputation," and indeed he turned out to be very accurate. He looked in his forties and he told me that his clairvoyant powers had dramatically increased when he was in his mid-thirties. He told me many things that I cannot reveal here, but regarding my condition he said, "You will wake up one morning and it will all be gone."

Another medium had said the same thing and it was what I prayed for night and day. During the session he also said, "I can see Portugal. Have you been to Portugal'?"

"No," I replied.

"Well you will be going there this summer—with the gentleman upstairs," he said. I just nodded, it seemed a bit optimistic, but Peter Lee had said the same thing.

Sometime later, when my condition had improved somewhat, I saw him again and he said, "When you first came here your face was white and taut. You looked like a tormented soul." He was right; I used to look in the mirror and the reflection staring back at me made me recoil in horror.

It was in that condition that I began to see my two newly acquired healers. The healer Peter Lee had recommended had contacted me the next day and I had made an appointment to see him the following week. But first I saw the lady healer who lived in Chelsea. She was now seventy but still very active in using her gift generously. Apart from having an open house on Wednesdays she visited hospitals etc, at the request of the patient's family. She didn't charge but you could leave a donation. Her assistant was a black gentleman called Bob. She, however, was rather a compulsive talker and it always took her a long time to get around to the actual healing. When she did get around to it I was required to sit on a stool while she stood behind me. Bob would sit on a stool in front of me and hold my hands. She would place her hands on my shoulders and immediately her right hand would begin to shake. She heals by working on the chakras—the energy centres of the body— and it seems to be very successful, especially for cancer victims. I didn't see many patients during my time with her, but I did see one lady who had it seems been cured of cancer of the bowel.

She said to me, "The specialists can find no trace of cancer now and I've only had a few healing sessions." I was very pleased for her. Francis had told me that the lady healer herself had had cancer on two occasions and about that she said, "When I asked, Why me? I heard a voice say, 'Why not you?" It seems that she goes into a trance and then speaks in a man's voice. When this happens people present say they can see a light above her head and others have said they can even see the face of her guide. Some of these happenings, that is, when her spirit guide talks through her, are recorded for she remembers nothing of it. One day they may be published.

The first time we went to her house she said, "I'm not a saint." Well we didn't think her to be a saint and neither did we expect her to be one. Alas, there have been very few real saints in the history of the whole world. Nevertheless she didn't endear herself to me by saying such things as, "You were pathetic when you first came." Also once snapping at me, "Be grateful that you're not in pain!" After all that I had been through you can imagine my feelings about those uncalled for remarks. It always astonishes me when you see someone with the most precious gift of all, the gift of healing, someone who should be and indeed very often professes to be more enlightened than the rest of us, are either blind to their own sad failings or do nothing to eradicate them. Arrogance, pride or jealousy are the usual causes. Bob, on the other hand, had none of those character defects and showed great sympathy towards my distress, whispering encouragement to me whenever he could. I am grateful to him for that.

The healer Peter Lee had recommended was, on the other hand, a professional healer who charged a fee. He was a short, bald man who, also unlike the lady healer, was a man of very few words. I used to be on a bed and he would hold his powerful hands over me. At the end of the session he would place his hands over mine about three inches apart and I could actually feel my hands tingling. "That's the good stuff," he would say. He was indeed a powerful healer. "I've been healing for forty years," he told me, "and I have a 75% success rate."

"Do you think my torment will eventually go?" I asked him.

"Oh yes," he replied, "I know when a person will not get better."

Once, when I lay on my stomach he held his hands over my back and my whole body shook. It was as if he had activated all the acupuncture points but, alas, when I tried to explain what it felt like he snapped back very disagreeably, "Oh, don't compare it with acupuncture." I diplomatically remained silent, knowing that healing was simply a routine job and profession to him. However, after a few weeks of seeing him he advised me to consult Dr Felix Mann saying, "He writes all the text books on acupuncture. I wouldn't send you to anyone but the best."

The last thing I wanted was to return to having acupuncture, but since he was such an expert I felt a consultation would do no harm. I found his name in the London directory and telephoned him. A lady answered, she turned out to be his wife. I asked for an appointment and then told her my problem—too much Ch'i in the head.

She replied, "You had better see him privately for a consultation because it's such an unusual case." I made an appointment to see him privately at his clinic near Harley Street, but he did hold open clinics on Tuesday mornings and Thursday afternoons when he charged half price.

He turned out to be a quietly spoken, very distinguished-looking gentleman, probably in his mid sixties. He was also a physician. I liked him; he was always very gracious to me.

He took down all the details of my predicament and at the end, although he didn't exactly refute that I had excess Ch'i in my head he said, "If I had to call it something, I would say you had tinnitus in the head." I just shook my head. However, he was aghast at the amount of acupuncture treatment I had had and thought I had been greatly overdone. "I've had people who have been overdone before but never in the head," he said. "But you should never have had harsh treatment, you are of a sensitive make up."

"What do you mean?" I asked.

"Well you're not a hefty, muscular male are you?" he answered, which illustrated the point he was making very clearly. I soon found out that he had a totally different approach to any other acupuncturist I had met. He held no brief with yin and yang philosophy and believes the process involves dermatone patches of skin that share nerve endings which are linked to internal organs. But the results of the treatment are the same, i.e. a needle in the foot can relieve migraine. He holds the needle in for about 10-15 seconds. He believes that balancing the energy flow is accomplished only with long experience of the body's intricate network of inner and outer relationships.

I was told to undress and put on a robe and when I had done so I sat on a chair and placed my right leg on another chair. He held the disposable needle in my right foot for about 15 seconds and then did the same with the back of my neck on the right side, because I had told him that the Ch'i almost always remained on the right side.

"If it works it will make the Ch'i go quicker," he said, "but if it doesn't work there is no point in wasting your money."

He refused to give me treatment once a week. He would only give me a treatment in a fortnight's time and then three weeks' time and so on, and when I asked him what treatment he was giving me he simply replied, "All I'm doing is relaxing the muscles in your neck. I'll write a letter to your GPs."

"What are you going to say to them?" I asked.

"I'll tell them that you've been greatly overdone," he replied.

That would be interesting I thought. They sneered at acupuncture and now the well-known Dr Felix Mann, an expert on acupuncture and a physician, would be writing to them.

Around July, the Ch'i began to stay mostly on the right side of my face, which was more bearable than in the head -it's not so sensitive, but it still caused me considerable distress. However, in one very rash moment we booked up to go to Portugal for two weeks. I was determined to enjoy it, but it proved to be premature. I had many very distressing days and nights and was required to take a sleeping pill on a few occasions. I remember one evening crying bitterly as we were on our way to a lovely restaurant that overlooked the sea. Nevertheless, on the whole I enjoyed it all.

We stayed in the Algarve but managed to travel to Lisbon and even Seville in Spain. Both Peter Lee and the African Seer had been correct and I prayed that their other predictions would eventually come to pass. I prayed constantly for the morning when I would wake up and it would all be gone. But that wasn't to be for a very long time to come. Even I had never envisaged how long it would take and the psychics had not been able to accurately foretell when it would eventually go, which was probably a good thing, for if in the beginning I had been told that I would have to suffer for many years to come my mind might not have been able to cope with it.

Meanwhile, the Ch'i continued to follow the same pattern. As I have stated, it stayed almost always on the right side of my head. One day it would sizzle all over the right side of my face, flitting about just like a pocket of electricity, one minute it was on my cheek, then my forehead, my nose, my lip, and even on my eyelid. Later on I used to feel it on the back of my neck. The following day it would die down somewhat and give me some relative peace and the tiniest fraction of Ch'i would have left my head going into some other part of the body where I wasn't aware of it. I could always tell the difference because it was altering all the time, but the process was so slow I despaired of it ever coming to an end.

At each stage, it still caused me considerable distress, even after three years. At the end when it had considerably thinned out, it seemed to be on the top of the skin, it was that superficial.

When I returned after my summer holiday abroad, I had no inclination to visit either of my two healers or Dr Felix Mann again, but I did promise him that I would let him know if and when the Ch'i finally left my head and I kept my promise.

Months passed and Christmas came and went. It was the third Christmas I had spent with the wretched Ch'i in my head and I prayed there would not be a fourth.

I was still attending the clinic in early 1989. The Ugandan gentleman had long since departed and instead I saw a young lady psychiatrist. The Ugandan gentleman had sensibly only concerned himself about my emotional state and not asked any further questions, and after a couple of months when my emotional state had definitely improved he said jubilantly, "We got you through it. You had practically given up," which was probably true.

The young lady, on the other hand, asked many questions about the Ch'i in my head, seemingly very interested. I was still taking 100 mg surmontil and living as normal a life as possible.

In the spring of 19891 began working seriously on the book, knocking it into some sort of shape, even having it typed out. But still there was no end in sight.

By the summer I felt well enough to cope with another holiday abroad and we booked up to go to Nice on the French Riviera. We both had a wonderful time and it proved less traumatic than the holiday I had had in Portugal the year before. The psychiatrist had said that she was leaving at the end of the summer and I would have another young lady psychiatrist when next I came, so I said to her, "You were the only doctor who believed me about the Ch'i in my head."

She looked puzzled, "What made you think I believed you?" she asked.

"Well you constantly questioned me about it," I replied in surprise.

"Only because it was important to you," she said smartly.

0I sighed. I really was naive. No doctor was ever likely to believe me. It was simply her method of trying to help me. After I returned from my holidays I dropped the 100 mg of surmontil I was taking to 50 mg and in September I went again to the clinic to see the new psychiatrist. She was obviously using the same kind of therapy and asked all about the Ch'i in my head. I told her that it was getting less and less all the time and tried to explain to her what it felt like, but she wanted to know how it all came about and when I mentioned the cube she wanted to know all about that too. However, she didn't seem to understand what I tried to tell her about the cube and asked many childlike questions like, "Were you attached to it?"

I told her the workstation was in Somerset and she could contact The Institute of Advanced Health Research if she wanted to know more about it, but she just stared blankly at me. She was convinced, I'm sure, that I was simply talking out of the top of my head.

"Are you depressed at the moment?" she asked.

"No, I'm fine," I said. "I'm not a depressed person. It was the torment I was in that caused my emotional collapse. I'm no longer in such torment."

"You can drop the 50 mg surmontil, but I'd like you to come just once more so that I can sign you off."

I went again to see her a few weeks later expecting it to be my last, but she surprised me by saying, "I want to help you. I want to take away what you've got in your head."

"How to you propose to do that?" I asked. "With medication," she replied.

"Oh! What medication?" I asked, as patiently as I could.

"Stelazine!" she replied.

I couldn't believe what I was hearing and said, "Oh I've heard about that drug, Miss Knight gave it to me."

"What did she say about it?" she asked sweetly.

"Well, she said that it was a very powerful drug which they gave to patients who were really mad and it helped to calm them down."

Her face flushed and she looked uncomfortable. "Why did she give you those?" she asked.

"I can't remember," I replied, "but they are still in the cabinet. I didn't take one of them."

It was true. She had given them to me on one of the very few occasions I had seen her at the surgery. She had refused to give me the anti-fungal drug nystatin, telling me I did not have Candida when in fact my whole body was affected by the illness. But she evidently had no qualms about giving me the drug stelazine which is used for severe mental disease to block electrical impulses in the brain, thus reducing abnormal behaviour and preventing delusions! How irresponsible can you get! And now this young lady psychiatrist was also suggesting that I took the same wretched drug when I clearly didn't need anything at all. But it was obvious to me that the fact that I was still talking about the Ch'i in my head and now the cube which she didn't understand meant to her that there was really something mentally wrong with me.

Even the psychiatrist at the hospital had put on record that there was nothing wrong with my mind, so why couldn't she accept that simple fact? It seemed I was back to square one! It was, indeed, very frustrating.

She continued to stare at me, so I went on to say as patiently as I could, "It has nothing to do with the mind," and added, "only a few acupuncturists ever believed me—those experts who knew that such a thing was possible." She flushed again but remained silent, so I went on, "I don't really know why it happened. It could have been entirely the fault of the acupuncturist whose treatment was, he admitted, very harsh. His treatment alone could have brought all the Ch'i into my head, but I think that being on the cube at the time, quite possibly, had a lot to do with it. It is hard to believe but the cube did have a devastating effect on my whole body, it ached tremendously—so much so I could hardly walk. It is designed to eradicate all the accumulated illnesses of a lifetime. However, when I realised something dreadful had gone wrong I asked to be taken off the cube immediately, but it was too late—the damage had been done and the consequences were terrible."

She listened to all I had to say but clearly she was out of her depth. She had no idea what I was talking about and even said afterwards, "Are you sure it doesn't feel like ants walking all over your head?"

"Quite sure," I replied sharply, knowing very well that it was one of the symptoms of the menopause, which she probably thought was the problem.

I didn't want to see her again because she was clearly wasting my time, but I agreed to see her once more, m a few months' time, when I would bring along with me the cube and all the information concerning it. Perhaps that would prove to her that they really did exist in fact and not in my imagination. However, when I told my husband what drug she offered me, he was extremely annoyed.

"I would have been furious," he said. Fortunately, I had been very placid, puffing it all down to her youth and inexperience. No doubt she meant well, but it was as if I was talking to an immature schoolgirl and I dread to think what utter rubbish they've got on my medical report. One day I hope to be able to read it for myself. At the time of writing, I hear they are trying to get a bill through Parliament which will enable me to do just that!

I never bothered to see her again. I regarded it as a complete waste of my time.

CHAPTER 16

Christmas 1989 came and went and I was obliged to spend yet another Christmas with the Ch'i still in my head—the fourth -which to me was unbelievable. There was enough Ch'i in my head to still cause me considerable distress and I took the odd sleeping pill to enable me to get some rest. Nevertheless, I was very much alive—I had survived! It was impossible to believe that all that happened because of what should have been a simple eye operation, but an operation that went so badly wrong. If someone had warned me that an infection was a possibility and that eye infections are so difficult to get rid of I would never have consented to the 'operation' in the first place. But the doctor was young and possibly inexperienced, and because of the amount of antibiotics I was prescribed, again without any warning as to the possible dangers, I developed Candida Albicans.

At the time, most doctors or specialists it seemed were totally unaware that such an illness even existed and, convinced that it was simply an 'emotional' state, I was sent to the inevitable psychiatrist. That of course, only made the situation even worse, for the drugs I was prescribed only suppressed the symptoms, leaving the Candida infection to flourish unchecked throughout my body for a couple of years.

I probably had one of the severest cases of Candida Albicans you could possibly have. Apart from the physical symptoms that I have described, I had terrible depression. I remember going one Saturday afternoon to the SAGB feeling frighteningly depressed and when the young gentleman healer put his hands over me he shrunk back in horror and said, "My God, I can actually feel the depression."

It was therefore, thank God, that there were just a few people in this country that knew about Candida Albicans and, as I have already stated,

I am forever grateful to the osteopath of the first Allergy Clinic I went to who correctly diagnosed my illness, which put me on the long road to recovery, and believe me it is a long road.

It was tragic, therefore, that because the Candida illness had so depleted my immune system I caught the severe virus that resulted in my having tinnitus in both ears. It was something I felt I really could not live with and in my desperation I had acupuncture whilst still being on the cube and the consequences of that was appalling. Whether being on the cube at the time had caused the Ch'i to rise into my head I shall probably never know or be able to prove, but no doubt there are a few people along the long line of disasters that I could possibly sue!

However, by March 1990,1 was so weary of still having to cope with the Ch'i sizzling on my face that I made an appointment to see an acupuncturist.

I had received treatment from her in the early days of Giovanni and Tina. I trusted her and regarded her as a very competent acupuncturist. I reasoned that a few sessions with her to give me a booster to try and earth the energy would do me no harm but at the last minute, I cancelled the appointment. I was worried in case she might alter the pattern. I knew it was getting less and less all the time so it was just a matter of accepting it and not getting unduly stressed until it finally left, which I knew would happen—sometime.

I managed somehow to do just that, which was a considerable achievement for me—I surprised even myself. However, towards the end of my ordeal I visited once again my local Spiritualist Church and during the evening of clairvoyance the gentleman medium pointed to me and said, "I want to talk to that lady."

I managed to mumble, "Thank you." I am always self-conscious when obliged to speak out in a crowded hall.

He went on, "All I'm getting from the spirits is, 'Tell her she has done well and we are very pleased with her.' They are giving you a deep red rose and the petals look like velvet."

Tears welled up into my eyes. I knew exactly what he meant.

At the beginning of June the Ch'i still hadn't completely disappeared from my head and one day, in frustration, I rushed to the cupboard where I keep the ash given to me by Lucas Ralli. He said Sai Baba had blessed it, so I plunged my finger into the small plastic container and then thrust my finger, which was coated with the ash, into my mouth and as I did so a date flashed before my eyes. Alas the Ch'i did not go on that day as I thought might happen, but hopefully something good will happen on that particular day another year.

During the most terrible time of my ordeal, when Dawn had seen me encased in a dark cave and could see no light, I had a dream in which I heard a voice say, "Christ will cure you." I never forgot it and on a day over nine years after the disaster happened I woke up to find at long last that the Ch'i had finally left my head. The relief was tremendous; it was heaven just to lie there in absolute peace.

Normally I would want to get up, or if compelled to lie down I would try and wander off into a trance thinking of all the most wonderful things which would completely obliterate the raging in my head or on my face where, for the last couple of years, it had stayed for most of the time, getting less and less as the years passed. But now, thank God, it has gone forever.

Dr Liu said it would never return and so did the lady medium and I'm sure it won't.

I remembered also at that time what that great healer Ted Fricker had said to me years before: "You're going to be fine," and indeed I was fine, albeit in need of some emotional peace and quiet.

The purpose for all the suffering as yet I do not know. If indeed it was Karma, as the lady medium said it was, then I don't regard Karma as a form of punishment but as an experience from which to learn.

Some time ago I read a book called *The Seth Material* by Jane Roberts Seth. A spirit entity speaking through Jane Roberts, had said, "Karma presents the opportunity for development. It enables the individual to enlarge understanding through experience, to fill the gaps of ignorance, to do what should be done. Free will is always involved." That seems to sum it up very nicely, for me at least. As for Candida Albicans—well I think the time has come for every doctor to recognise and accept that it is a real and devastating illness. Certainly there is more publicity given to it in the media. However, once the infection has taken a hold, the journey back to health is not an easy one and I doubt whether the average OP will be able to cope with it. The process is long and extremely complicated, involving anti-fungal drugs, a good bowel flora, a rigid yeast free diet, many supplements of vitamins and minerals etc and above all, for the patient, dedication. I have gone through it and I know it is not an easy task, but the return to health is the reward for all the patience and resolve. I once belonged to the Candida Albicans Advice Group and they provide a list of doctors who specialise in treating that particular illness, but unfortunately privately only. And as for the people who ridicule the idea that there is such a thing as a force or energy that runs through the body, well all I can say is that I have experienced what it is like to have a head full of a force which the Chinese have always known about—they call it Ch'i. Recently I read a book called *Kind to Mind* by Betty Shine. She is a clairvoyant diagnostic healer and when healing she works on the energy field. She writes in her book that she can see what looks like tubes running through the body corresponding to the meridian lines of the Chinese acupuncture—the energy lines. And another thing I found interesting in her book was the fact that during healing she and the patient feel a sensation like strands of spider's web on their faces. She says she can see them trying to remove it from their face. She calls it an uncanny phenomenon and the only explanation she has for it is that it is some sort of floating energy.

How right she is, for I have experienced that so-called phenomenon over and over again, especially towards the end when the Ch'i had considerably thinned out and spread, as it often did, over my face. I myself used the same description when trying to explain to my husband what it felt like—a spider's web on my face. I, too, often put my hands to my face to try and remove it, but alas mine did not go miraculously but in its own time. However, now it has gone forever and as one kind medium put it, "Afterwards you will never look back."

God Bless.

Dr Felix Mann has recently written a book called *Reinventing Acupuncture—A New Concept of Ancient Medicine*. In a newspaper article he says, "When I first started, most of my colleagues thought I was fit only for the loony bin. I've now trained over a thousand doctors myself and the courses are getting more popular. It's now time to get rid of the myths and rubbish surrounding the subject and put acupuncture in the proper scientific footing where it belongs."

With my experience of Ch'i that has gone completely out of its proper place I think I could significantly add something to the scientific aspect of the subject.

THE END